SpringerBriefs in Bioengineering

T0234487

More information about this series at http://www.springer.com/series/10280

Yunfeng Wu

Knee Joint Vibroarthrographic Signal Processing and Analysis

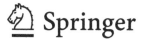

Yunfeng Wu
School of Information Science and Technology
Xiamen University
Xiamen, Fujian, China

ISSN 2193-097X   ISSN 2193-0988   (electronic)
SpringerBriefs in Bioengineering
ISBN 978-3-662-44283-8   ISBN 978-3-662-44284-5   (eBook)
DOI 10.1007/978-3-662-44284-5

Library of Congress Control Number: 2014959278

Springer Heidelberg New York Dordrecht London

Printed on acid-free paper

Springer-Verlag GmbH Berlin Heidelberg is part of Springer Science+Business Media (www.springer.
com)

To my grandparents: Weiqing Wu, Meihui Su;
Shaowen Xiong, Xiuying Ruan

Yunfeng Wu

Preface

The knee plays an important role in human locomotion activities and daily performance. However, the knee joint often suffers from different inflammations and impact trauma such as osteoarthritis, tears of meniscus, and cartilage disorders. Vibration arthrometry is a noninvasive technique which has high potential for effective detection of knee pathology in routine examinations. This book provides a systematical description on the vibroarthrograpy methodology, along with the recent advances in vibroarthrographic signal preprocessing, feature analysis, and pattern classification. The overall context of the book is composed of five chapters.

Chapter 1 presents knee anatomy, together with the descriptions of joint structures in detail. The text introduces knee biomechanics and different types of knee joint disorders. An overview of knee joint pathology detection methods, such as X-ray imaging, computed tomography, magnetic resonance imaging, ultrasonography, optical coherence tomography, arthroscopy, and vibroarthrography, is given in the chapter as well.

Chapter 2 provides the flowchart that shows the entire procedures of knee joint vibroarthrographic signal analysis. The chapter concentrates on the instrument settings and experiment protocol for signal acquisition, as well as the artifact removal in the signal preprocessing. The text describes several signal processing methods to eliminate the baseline wander, random noise, and muscle contraction interference.

Chapter 3 discusses the vibroarthrographic signal processing and analysis approaches in time and frequency domains. The spatiotemporal processing methods contain the temporal waveform analysis, adaptive segmentations, and time-variant signal fluctuation or complexity analysis. The frequency and time-frequency analysis based on Fourier transform and matching pursuit decomposition are also provided with the detailed mathematical representations. The chapter also reviews the recent development of statistical analysis for vibroarthrographic signal feature extraction.

Chapter 4 first presents the advantages of feature selection and dimensionality reduction for signal pattern analysis. Then, the chapter introduces a few machine learning paradigms for vibroarthrographic signal classifications, including the

Fisher's linear discriminant analysis, radial basis function network, support vector machines, Bayesian decision rule, and multiple classifier fusion systems. The chapter also summarizes and compares the diagnostic results and key findings of several previous studies on vibroarthrographic signal classifications.

Chapter 5 concludes the book with a short review of the cutting-edge technologies for knee pathology diagnosis, and then summarizes the state-of-the-art methods for vibroarthrographic signal analysis. The chapter ends with a discussion on some interesting topics and challenges for future research.

Xiamen, Fujian, China   Yunfeng Wu

Acknowledgements

I would like to take this opportunity to express my gratitude to Prof. Rangaraj M. Rangayyan, who supervised my PhD dissertation on this research topic, and Prof. Sridhar Krishnan, who collaborated with me in the field of biomedical signal analysis. I also thank the members of my research group: Ms. Suxian Cai, Ms. Shanshan Yang, Ms. Xin Luo, Mr. Kaizhi Liu, Mr. Lei Shi, Ms. Fang Zheng, Mr. Meng Lu, Ms. Pinnan Chen, and Prof. Meihong Wu, for their diligent work and hearty contributions on the research projects. Finally, I acknowledge the research grants supported by the National Natural Science Foundation of China (grant no. 81101115), the Fundamental Research Funds for the Central Universities of China (grant no. 2010121061), and the Program for New Century Excellent Talents in Fujian Province University.

Contents

Abbreviations

ACL	Anterior cruciate ligament
AEA	Averaged envelope amplitude
AR	Autoregressive
CMP	Chondromalacia patellae
CT	Computed tomography
CV	Coefficient of variation
DFA	Detrended fluctuation analysis
ECG	Electrocardiogram
EEG	Electroencephalogram
EEMD	Ensemble empirical mode decomposition
EMD	Empirical mode decomposition
EMG	Electromyogram
EP	Energy parameter
ESP	Energy spread parameter
FBLP	Forward-backward linear prediction
FD	Fractal dimension
FF	Form factor
FFT	Fast Fourier transform
FLDA	Fisher's linear discriminant analysis
FP	Frequency parameter
FSI	Fractal scaling index
FSP	Frequency spread parameter
HE	Hurst exponent
Hz	Hertz
IMF	Intrinsic mode function
KLD	Kullback-Leibler divergence
KU	Kurtosis
LCL	Lateral collateral ligament
LDA	Local discriminant analysis
LDB	Local discriminant bases

LMS	Least mean squares
LOO	Leave one out
LS-SVM	Least-squares support vector machine
MCI	Muscle contraction interference
MCL	Medial collateral ligament
MDP	Power and median frequency
MLP	Multilayer perceptron
MP	Matching pursuit
MRI	Magnetic resonance imaging
ms	Millisecond
MSE	Mean-squared error
NTKP	Normal total knee replacement
OA	Osteoarthritis
OCT	Optical coherence tomography
PCL	Posterior cruciate ligament
PDF	Probability density function
PSD	Power spectral density
RBFN	Radial basis function network
RLS	Recursive least-squares
ROC	Receiver operating characteristics
SBS	Sequential backward selection
SD	Standard deviation
sec	Second
SED	Squared Euclidean distance
SFS	Sequential forward selection
SNR	Signal-to-noise ratio
SK	Skewness
STFT	Short-time Fourier transform
SVD	Singular value decomposition
SVM	Support vector machine
TFD	Time-frequency distribution
VAG	Vibroarthrography or vibroarthrographic
VMG	Vibromyogram

Chapter 1
Introduction

Abstract This chapter describes the knee joint anatomy in the human body, along with its biomechanical behaviors. The text presents the structures of femoropatellar, medial and lateral femorotibial articulations. The chapter also provides an overview of different types of knee joint disorders and the related medical diagnosis methods.

1.1 Knee Joint Anatomy

The knee joint is the largest and most complicated joint that connects the thigh and shank in the human body [21]. As shown in Fig. 1.1, the knee includes three articulating bones, i.e., the femur (thighbone), patella (knee cap), and the tibia (shinbone), in the lower extremity of the body. The femur, also called the thighbone, is the longest and strongest bone in the body. The two round protuberances at the end of the femur are called femoral condyles. These femoral condyles form a groove named the patellofemoral groove. The patella glides along the bottom front surface of the femur between the femoral condyles. The function of the patella is to protect the knee by relieving frictions between the cartilages and muscles, when the knee performs bending motions. Tibia is commonly called the shinbone which helps stabilize the knee. Two crescent-shaped menisci are attached at the top of the tibia. The fibula next to the tibia also supports the joint stability, but it is not involved with the joint capsule.

The knee joint consists of three functional compartments [82]: the patellofemoral articulation located between the patella and the femur, the lateral femorotibial articulation, and the medial femorotibial articulation. The patellofemoral articulation is a synovial gliding joint, and the two femorotibial articulations between the femur and the tibia are synovial hinge joints [64].

The knee joint is an intricate synovial joint because the joint is bathed in synovial fluid, which is secreted by a synovial membrane [57]. The articular surface of the joint is surrounded by a synovial capsule. The synovial membrane located in the inner layer of the capsule produces the synovial fluid, which consists of hyaluronic acid, lubricin, proteinases, and collagenases. The synovial fluid in the knee joint helps lubricate and cushion the joint without any friction in motions.

© The Author(s) 2015
Y. Wu, *Knee Joint Vibroarthrographic Signal Processing and Analysis*,
SpringerBriefs in Bioengineering, DOI 10.1007/978-3-662-44284-5_1

1

Fig. 1.1 Schematic
representations of a knee joint

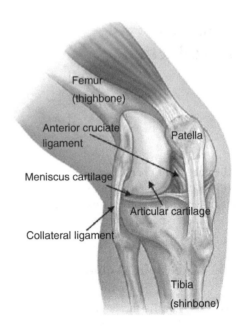

1.1.1 Ligaments

Ligaments are strong fibrous tissue bands that attach the knee bones with each other.
There are four major ligaments providing strength and stability to the human knee.
The medial collateral ligament (MCL) attaches the medial side of the femur to the
medial side of the tibia, and protects the normal-range sideways motion from a
valgus stress [77]. The lateral collateral ligament (LCL) attaches the lateral side
of the femur to the lateral side of the fibula, and limits the lateral-side sliding from
a varus stress [77].

The anterior and posterior cruciate ligaments are two crisscross intracapsular
ligaments in the center of the knee joint. The anterior cruciate ligament (ACL)
lies deep within the notch of the distal femur (see Fig. 1.1). Its function is to
resist anterior translation and medial rotation of the tibia relative to the femur.
The posterior cruciate ligament (PCL) connects the posterior intercondylar area of
the tibia to the medial condyle of the femur. The PCL is able to prevent posterior
displacement of the tibia, in relation to the femur.

1.1.2 Menisci

The meniscus are a pair of crescent-shaped pads of fibrocartilaginous structures,
as shown in Fig. 1.2. The lateral and medial menisci of the knee joint lie on the
articular surface of the tibia. These two shock-absorbing cartilages are able to

Fig. 1.2 Transverse view of
the lateral and medial menisci
in the knee joint

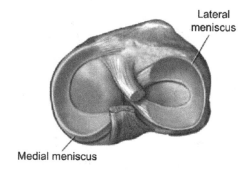

Lateral
meniscus

Medial meniscus

provide structural integrity to the knee when it undergoes tension and torsion, and
can also disperse the load and reduce friction over the articular surfaces of the tibia
and femur in the knee joint.

1.1.3   Articular Cartilage

The articular surfaces of the knee joint are the large curved condyles of the femur,
the flattened condyles (medial and lateral plateaus) of the tibia, and the facets of the
patella [50]. Like all the major joints of the human body, the articular surfaces of
the knee joint are covered by cartilage. In addition to the meniscus, the other type
of cartilage that pads the ends of the articulation bones in the knee is called articular
cartilage. The articular cartilage is a type of smooth and white tissue in the knee
joint, and is composed of a solid matrix (20–30 % by wet weight) and synovial fluid
(70–80 % by wet weight). The solid matrix consists primarily of type II collagen
and aggrecan, the latter of which is referred to as a chondroitin and keratan sulfate
proteoglycan [90]. Articular cartilage is able to cushion the impact of knee during
locomotion and bounce activities [90].

1.2   Biomechanics of the Knee

The knee permits a typical rolling-gliding mechanism of flexion and extension with
its six degrees of freedom (three in translation and three in rotation). The translations
of the knee take place on the anterior-posterior, medial-lateral, and proximal-
distal axes. The rotational motion consists of flexion-extension and internal-external
rotation. In general, the knee rotation is associated with some degree of translation,
and vice versa, because the femur and menisci move over the tibia during rotation,
while the femur rolls and glides over the menisci during extension-flexion [57].
When the knee is fully extended, the tibia and femur are locked in place, so that they
will not become unlocked until flexion is initiated [32]. When the knee is flexed,

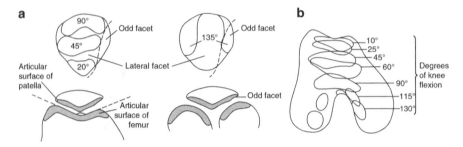

Fig. 1.3 Patellar contact areas during the patellofemoral articulation: (**a**) patellar cartilage contact facets; (**b**) contact areas over the articular surface of the femur at different degrees of the knee flexion

the contact areas of the patellofemoral articulation migrate progressively upward, involving both the medial and lateral facets of the patella from approximately 20° of flexion [29] (see Fig. 1.3). At 90° of knee flexion, the patellofemoral contact areas engage the upper pole of the patella. At about 120°–135° of flexion, the patellar odd facet articulates with the lateral margin of the medial femoral condyle.

1.3 Knee Joint Disorders

The knee joint supports nearly the entire weight of the human body, and also provides bending motion during walking. It is most vulnerable both to injury and the development of osteoarthritis (OA) in the human body [86]. In daily activities such as normal walking or running, the knee can tolerate moderate stress without significant injury. But the knee lacks support to withstand rotational forces and other types of physical trauma, such that it is still often injured in strenuous exercises [28, 86].

The ACL tears usually occur when landing or performing pivoting exercises, especially for athletes. The patellar tendon and the hamstrings tendon are commonly used as source tissues for autograft in the ACL reconstruction surgery. The PCL injuries are mainly caused when the tibia is displaced posterior to the femur during hyperflexion or hyperextension of the knee joint [14]. The MCL is usually injured as a result of a valgus stress to a slightly bent knee, and such a injury mostly occurs in skiing sports. On the other hand, the varus stress across the knee may lead to the LCL injuries.

There are two main types of meniscus injuries: acute tears and chronic tears. Sports activities or trauma may lead to meniscal acute tears with different shapes and sizes. Chronic tears are often the result of severe overload on the knee joint. Acute tears of meniscus could be treated with surgical repair, and chronic tears should be controlled by physical therapy or anti-inflammatory medications.

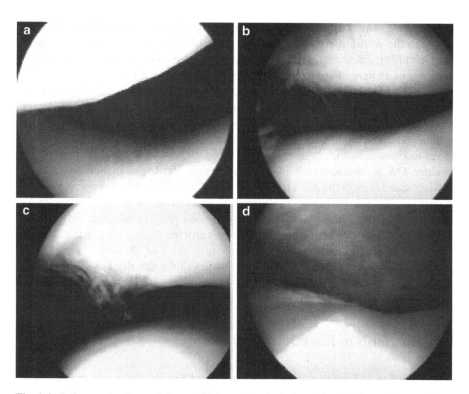

Fig. 1.4 Arthroscopic views of the patellofemoral articulation: (**a**) normal cartilage surfaces; (**b**) chondromalacia Grade II at the patella; (**c**) chondromalacia Grade III at the patella; (**d**) chondromalacia Grade IV at the patella and the femur; the bones are exposed. The undersurface of patella is at the top and the femoral condyle is at the bottom (Reprinted with permission from Ref. [90]. © 2010 Begell House)

Chondromalacia of the patella is the result common to a wide variety of unusual trauma [61], with the syndrome of pain over the posterior patellar cartilage surface [30]. Chondromalacia patellae has been considered to be a precursor of OA [88]. In the degenerative course of arthritis with aging, chondromalacia patellae is initially characterized by swelling with superabundant water content and softening due to the reduction of proteoglycan [33]. According to the severity of the lesions, the classification of chondromalacia patellae is commonly defined by four progressive stages in terms of Grade I–IV [60], as shown in Fig. 1.4.

Impact trauma to the articular cartilage or the menisci may cause deterioration of articular surfaces or secondary OA [20, 51, 63]. Nontraumatic conditions of the knee could also lead to OA. With the degeneration of the patellofemoral compartment, loss of cartilage may be localized on the medial and lateral articular surfaces of the patella. Because the medial meniscus is firmly attached to the tibial collateral ligament, it is more likely to be torn due to traumatic rupture than the lateral meniscus, which is smaller in shape and not attached to the lateral ligament [75].

Knee OA, which affects 1,770 men and 2,693 women out of every 100,000 people in the world, is the most common form of inflammation in a degenerative knee joint [79]. Epidemiological studies [25, 26] have reported that 19 % of people at the age of 45 have radiographic evidence of knee OA, which increases to 27 % for people aged 63–69 years, and to 44 % for people older than 80 years. The incidence of knee OA is higher in females than in males and increases with age, while not being limited to the elderly. A significant proportion of OA cases is associated with trauma and obesity; however, a large number of OA cases are idiopathic (with an as-yet-unknown cause).

Knee OA is characterized by the degenerative changes in bones, articular cartilages, and the soft tissues. The disease may affect any of the three compartments of the knee: medial, lateral, or patellofemoral articulation. Articular cartilage lacks the vascular supply and is deficient of innervation [86]. In addition, progressive thinning of articular surfaces also occurs due to cartilage degeneration in the affected knee joint. Since knee OA is the most common cause of rheumatic complaints, effective diagnostic techniques at the early stages of the OA disease are important and have high potential for clinical control of the course of cartilage degeneration.

1.4 Diagnosis of Knee Joint Pathology

Early detection of knee joint pathology can help clinicians apply appropriate thera-peutical or surgical procedures to control the degenerative process of arthritis [28]. Besides the general clinical examination, imaging-based techniques, arthroscopy, and vibroarthrography (VAG) [64] can be used for the diagnosis of cartilage pathol-ogy. Imaging techniques, such as X-ray, computed tomography (CT), magnetic resonance (MR) imaging, ultrasonography, optical coherence tomography, and the vibroarthrography can be used for noninvasive assessment of knee joint disorders. Arthroscopy is a semi-invasive surgical procedure for diagnosis and treatment of knee joint pathology.

1.4.1 X-Ray Imaging

Digital radiography cannot provide a direct appreciation of the status of the articular cartilage, because the cartilage is not visible on X-ray images [10]. It is, therefore, vital to demonstrate precisely the joint space of the knee [85]. Joint space narrowing, osteophytes, and subchondral bone sclerosis are the main signs of knee OA on X-ray images [3]. Joint space narrowing can reflect cartilage thickness on X-ray images; osteophytes indicate marginal bone reaction proportional to the loss of cartilaginous substance; and subchondral bone reactions or condensation are associated with

Fig. 1.5 Sagittal digital
X-ray image of left knee
joint: degenerative disorders
on the cartilage surfaces, joint
space narrowing, and
calcification upon the patellar
bursae (75-years-old male)

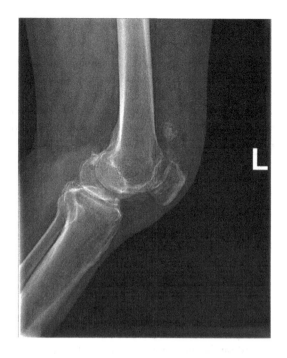

the overlying fibrocartilaginous damage [27]. Figure 1.5 displays a sagittal X-ray
image of a 75-year-old male patient with degenerative disorders on the cartilage
surfaces, joint space narrowing, and calcification upon the patellar bursae. With
a combination of three views (frontal view, lateral view, and tangential view),
the radiologist can perform a relatively reliable and reproducible analysis of the
patellofemoral compartment [12]. Although a frontal view of the knee may be
helpful in planning surgery, the ideal radiographic examination of the knee requires
proper inclination and alignment of the X-ray beam, which have to be carefully
performed under radioscopic control. With regards to joint space narrowing, the
only specific radiographical sign that corresponds exactly to the loss of cartilage, is
not readily evident on X-ray images. Thus, conventional radiography based on atlas
classifications has some difficulties in the diagnosis of pre-arthritis [10]. Based upon
the results of clinical examination and X-ray images, patients are typically graded
according to the Kellgren-Lawrence scale [2, 37]. The scale provides five grades
in the range 0–4, with grades 0 and 1 indicating normal and doubtful cases; 2 and
3 indicating evidence of the presence of mild and moderate OA; and 4 indicating
evidence of severe OA. Since knee OA at early stages may not show clearly evident
features on the standard X-ray images obtained in an initial exam, patients with
complaints related to the knee joint and X-ray images with Kellgren-Lawrence
grades of 0 and 1 may be advised further examination via other imaging or detection
techniques.

1.4.2 Computed Tomography

CT is commonly used as a supplement to conventional arthrography. It is more effective in the assessment of bone injuries rather than soft tissues. CT scanning with iodized articular injection can provide excellent visualization of the intra-articular structures, contours of the condyles, and tibial plateau surfaces [1]. Such a technology visualizes the degree of the distal femur fractures, along with the stress fractures of the tibial plateau and proximal fibula in the knee joint [1]. The drawback of CT evaluation is that this technique can detect only gross defects in the knee [13]. In addition, CT fails to characterize the functional integrity of cartilage, in terms of softening, stiffness, or fissuring.

1.4.3 Ultrasonography

Ultrasound imaging is extremely sensitive in the detection of soft tissue changes in the osteoarthritic joints, and it helps rheumatologists establish the guidelines for assessment of abnormalities of articular cartilage, bony cortex and synovial tissue [56]. The setting of ultrasound equipment and scanning guidelines greatly depend on the anatomic site and the tissue examined [4]. The ultrasonic frequency should be chosen higher than 13 MHz for the optimal visualization of cartilage, and lower than 10 MHz for hip joint assessment [56]. To assess the OA condition, the multiplanar scanning technique on two or more perpendicular scanning planes is required. Ultrasound imaging can show minute changes of soft tissues, tendons, ligaments, synovial recesses, bursae, cartilage, and peripheral conditions of the menisci. However, the ultrasonic visualization of articular cartilage is limited by the acoustic windows, whose width is determined by the anatomy of the joint tested, because the ultrasound beam is not able to penetrate bony cortex [56].

1.4.4 Magnetic Resonance Imaging

MR imaging is sensitive to defects of articular cartilage surfaces [11]. The choice of the type of sequence (T1-, T2-, or proton density-weighted imaging) is important to obtain good image contrast, in order to facilitate discrimination between cartilage and synovial fluid [8, 76]. Eckstein et al. [22, 23] demonstrated that MR imaging could be used for repeatable determination of articular cartilage thickness, and also reported that topographical maps obtained from MR images may assist in the characterization of in vivo orthopaedic conditions. MR imaging can also detect chondromalacia, which cannot be visualized by X-ray or CT imaging. van Leersum et al. [84] reported that T2-weighted conventional and fast spin-echo sequences with fat suppression are more accurate than proton density, T1-weighted, and gradient-echo sequences in grading chondromalacia. However, they also admitted that good histologic and macroscopic correlation could only be seen in severe grades of chondromalacia, and that MR imaging was not successful in the detection of early grades of chondromalacia [84]. Generally speaking, the MR imaging technique is still developing, and routine imaging of human joints is not fully established in clinical practice (Figs. 1.6 and 1.7).

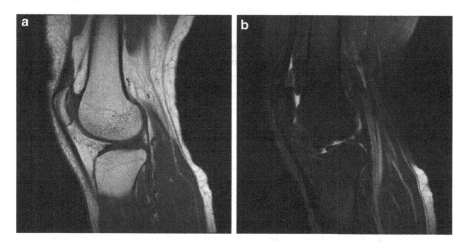

Fig. 1.6 Sagittal views of the osteochondritis dissecans in the knee joint (46-years-old female): (**a**) T1-weighted MR image; (**b**) T2-weighted MR image

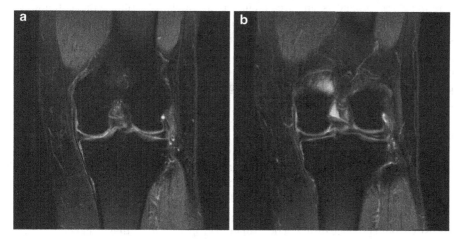

Fig. 1.7 Coronal T2-weighted MR sequence of the meniscus injuries in the left knee joint (39-years-old female): (**a**) medial meniscus injury (Grade II); (**b**) lateral meniscus injury (Grade II–III)

1.4.5 Optical Coherence Tomography

As a recently developed infrared-based imaging technique, optical coherence tomography (OCT) also demonstrated some merits in osteoarthritis detection, by providing in vivo cartilage images at a resolution of micrometers [48, 70]. The OCT generates the infrared light that is split into a sample and a reference arm. The infrared light reflecting back from the sample is combined with the light from the reference arm mirror [70]. The intensity of interference is measured using the low-coherence interferometry method. When the infrared beam is scanned across the tissue surface, three-dimensional images can be produced to interpret the microstructure of the tissue [70]. Recently, preliminary studies [31, 48] using the polarization-sensitivity OCT imaging in vivo and in vitro of articular cartilage have successfully demonstrated the potential merits in the assessment of osteoarthritic knees. However, the standardized OCT scanning guidelines based on more clinical trials are necessary to establish for effective monitoring of osteoarthritis progression.

1.4.6 Arthroscopy

Arthroscopy is commonly performed as a semi-invasive surgical procedure [49]. The surgeon is able to inspect the interior of a knee with an arthroscope that can be inserted into the joint through a small incision. Arthroscopy has emerged as the "gold standard" for relatively low-risk assessment of joint surfaces to determine the prognosis and treatment for a variety of orthopaedic conditions [34]. Before the advent of arthroscopy and arthroscopic surgery, patients having surgery for a torn ACL required several months of rehabilitation [53]. Although arthroscopy is an excellent tool for the assessment of cartilaginous losses and classification of chondromalacia lesions [49], the procedure cannot be applied to patients whose knees are in a highly degenerated state due to OA, ligamentous instability, meniscectomy, or patellectomy [19]. In addition, arthroscopy is not well-suited for repeated assessment of patients over time, due to its semi-invasive nature and anaesthesia requirements [74].

Recent studies [41, 47] reported that the early onset of cartilage degeneration may occur prior to any visible change on the articular surface. Quantitative mechanical evaluation using a handheld indentation probe during knee arthroscopy has been introduced to detect the irreversible early-degenerative changes in articular cartilage tissue [41, 47]. The recent related work suggested that the indenter geometry and its porosity would produce different deformation properties in cartilage, and may affect the precise evaluation of cartilage degeneration [47].

1.4.7   Vibroarthrography

During normal knee motions, both the intra- and extra-articular components may produce vibrations or sounds as they pass over one another [38, 87]. The knee joint sound, which is emitted from a knee joint in the course of flexion or extension, is referred to as the vibroarthrographic (VAG) signal [28, 64].

The diagnostic potential of knee joint sounds in noninvasive detection of articular cartilage disorders was first reported by Blodgett [7] in 1902. The first graphical recording of knee joint sounds by means of a microphone was implemented by Erb [24] in 1933. After that, with the investigations conducted by Steindler [78], Peylan [62], and Chu et al. [15–18], joint auscultation setup and configuration have become more and more sophisticated. However, microphone-based techniques are not well-suited for clinical detection of joint disorders, because a microphone-based joint auscultation system has a limited frequency response in the audible range, and its sensitivity is commonly diminished by artifacts such as ambient noise and skin friction.

Mollan et al. [54, 55] reported that appropriate choice or design of the sensor was essential to solve the detection problem, and they proposed using an accelerometer, instead of a microphone, to measure joint vibrations or sounds. Later, Kernohan et al. [38, 39] developed the techniques of vibration arthrometry; they started with a pilot study to detect congenital hip dislocation in an infant group, and then extended vibration arthrometry to diagnose meniscal lesions and to assess the mechanical characteristics of articular cartilage. Their studies demonstrated that the knee joint VAG signals recorded from subjects with meniscal injuries would exhibit distinct patterns [38]. Vibration arthrometry was also used by McCoy et al. [52] before and after corrective surgery, in an attempt to obtain an objective assessment of the efficacy of arthroscopic surgery. They observed that the VAG signals recorded from some patients who had undergone meniscal resection showed a significant reduction in energy, in comparison with the preoperative signals [52]. Physiological patellofemoral crepitus is referred to as a series of transients or vibration pulses generated between the patellar and femoral surfaces, typically observed when the normal knee is flexed or extended at 3° per second [6]. Patellofemoral crepitus contains two overlapping components. Beverland et al. [5] reported that the inherent component can be estimated using a weighted-mean calculation method, and the repetition component can be estimated in the time domain by a cross-over method. Patellofemoral crepitus has been considered to be useful for noninvasive assessment of the integrity of the patellofemoral articulation [35, 46].

From the 1990s, with the development of advanced techniques for digital signal processing and machine learning, significant progress has been made in the measurement and analysis of VAG signals [9, 36, 40, 42–45, 58, 59, 65–69, 71–73, 80, 81, 83, 89, 91–93]. The following chapters present a review of recent progress in the area of knee joint VAG signal analysis, together with the state-of-the-art pattern classification tools for screening knee joint disorders.

References

1. Ahn JM, El-Khoury GY (2006) Computed tomography of knee injuries. Imaging Decis MRI 10(1):14–23
2. Altman RD (2004) Measurement of structure (disease) modification in osteoarthritis. Osteoarthr Cartil 12(Suppl 1):69–76
3. Altman RD, Fries JF, Bloch DA, Carstensm J, DerekMb TC, Genant H, Gofton P, Groth H, Mcshane DJ, Murphy WA, Sharp JT, Spitz P, Williams CA, Wolfe F (1987) Radiographic assessment of progression in osteoarthritis. Arthritis Rheum 30(11):1214–1225
4. Backhaus M, Burmester GR, Gerber T, Grassi W, Machold KP, Swen WA, Wakefield RJ, Manger B (2001) Guidelines for musculoskeletal ultrasound in rheumatology. Ann Rheum Dis 60(7):641–649
5. Beverland DE, Kernohan WG, Mollan RAB (1985) Problems in the analysis of vibration emission from the patello-femoral joint. Med Biol Eng Comput 23(Suppl 2):1253–1254
6. Beverland DE, Kernohan WG, Mollan RAB (1985) What is physiological patello-femoral crepitus? Med Biol Eng Comput 23(Suppl 2):1249–1250
7. Blodgett WE (1902) Auscultation of the knee joint. Boston Med Surg J 146(3):63–66
8. Bredella MA, Tirman PF, Peterfy CG, Zarlingo M, Feller JF, Bost FW, Belzer JP, Wischer TK, Genant HK (1999) Accuracy of T2-weighted fast spin-echo MR imaging with fat saturation in detecting cartilage defects in the knee: comparison with arthroscopy in 130 patients. Am J Roentgenol 172(4):1073–1080
9. Cai S, Yang S, Zheng F, Lu M, Wu Y, Krishnan S (2013) Knee joint vibration signal analysis with matching pursuit decomposition and dynamic weighted classifier fusion. Comput Math Methods Med 2013:Article ID 904267
10. Carrillon Y (2008) Imaging knee osteoarthritis. In: Bonnin M, Chambat P (eds) Osteoarthritis of the knee. Springer, Paris, pp 3–14
11. Cashman PMM, Kitney RI, Gariba MA, Carter ME (2002) Automated techniques for visualization and mapping of articular cartilage in MR images of the osteoarthritic knee: a base technique for the assessment of microdamage and submicro damage. IEEE Trans Nanobiosci 1(1):42–51
12. Chaisson CE, Gale DR, Gale E, Kazis L, Skinner K, Felson DT (2000) Detecting radiographic knee osteoarthritis: what combination of views is optimal? Rheumatology 39(11):1218–1221
13. Chan WP, Lang P, Stevens MP, Sack K, Majumdar S, Stoller DW, Basch C, Genant HK (1991) Osteoarthritis of the knee: comparison of radiography, CT, and MR imaging to assess extent and severity. Am J Roentgenol 157(4):799–806
14. Chandrasekaran S, Ma D, Scarvell JM, Woods KR, Smith PN (2012) A review of the anatomical, biomechanical and kinematic findings of posterior cruciate ligament injury with respect to non-operative management. The Knee 19(6):738–745
15. Chu ML, Gradisar IA, Railey MR, Bowling GF (1976) Detection of knee joint diseases using acoustical pattern recognition technique. J Biomech 9:111–114
16. Chu ML, Gradisar IA, Railey MR, Bowling GF (1976) An electro-acoustical technique for the detection of knee joint noise. Med Res Eng 12(1):1820
17. Chu ML, Gradisar IA, Mostardi R (1978) A noninvasive electroacoustical evalution technique of cartilage damage in pathological knee joints. Med Biol Eng Comput 16:437–442
18. Chu ML, Gradisar IA, Zavodney LD (1978) Possible clinical application of a noninvasive monitoring technique of cartilage damage in pathological knee joints. J Clin Eng 3(1):19–27
19. Dandy DJ (1987) Arthroscopic management of the knee. Churchill Livingstone, New York
20. Dejour D, Vasconcelos W, Tavernier T (2008) Patellofemoral osteoarthritis. In: Bonnin M, Chambat P (eds) Osteoarthritis of the knee. Springer, Paris, pp 15–33
21. Diab M (1999) Lexicon of orthopaedic etymology. Harwood Academic, Newark
22. Eckstein F, Adam C, Sittek H, Becker C, Milz S, Schulte E, Reiser M, Putz R (1997) Non-invasive determination of cartilage thickness throughout joint surfaces using magnetic resonance imaging. J Biomech 30(3):285–289

23. Eckstein F, Westhoff J, Sittek H, Maag KP, Haubner M, Faber S, Englmeier KH, Reiser M (1998) In vivo reproducibility of three-dimensional cartilage volume and thickness measurements with MR imaging. Am J Roentgenol 170(3):593–597

24. Erb KH (1933) Über die möglichkeit der registrierung von gelenkgeräuschen. Deutsche Zeitschrift für Chirurgie 241:237–245

25. Felson DT (1990) The epidemiology of knee osteoarthritis: results from the Framingham osteoarthritis study. Semin Arthritis Rheumatol 20(3 Suppl 1):42–50

26. Felson DT, Zhang Y, Hannan MT, Naimark A, Weissman BN, Aliabadi P, Levy D (1995) The incidence and natural history of knee osteoarthritis in the elderly: the Framingham osteoarthritis study. Arthritis Rheum 38(10):1500–1505

27. Fife RS, Brandt KD, Braunstein EM, Katz BP, Shelbourne KD, Kalasinski LA, Ryan S (1991) Relationship between arthroscopic evidence of cartilage damage and radiographic evidence of joint space narrowing in early osteoarthritis of the knee. Arthritis Rheum 34(4):377–382

28. Frank CB, Rangayyan RM, Bell GD (1990) Analysis of knee sound signals for non-invasive diagnosis of cartilage pathology. IEEE Eng Med Biol Mag 9(1):65–68

29. Goodfellow J, Hungerford DS, Zindel M (1976) Patello-femoral joint mechanics and pathology, Part 1: functional anatomy of the patello-femoral joint. J Bone Jt Surg Br Vol 58-B(3):287–290

30. Goodfellow J, Hungerford DS, Woods C (1976) Patello-femoral joint mechanics and pathology, Part 2: chondromalacia patellae. J Bone Jt Surg Br Vol 58-B(3):291–299

31. Herrmann JM, Pitris C, Bouma BE, Boppart SA, Jesser CA, Stamper DL, Fujimoto JG, Brezinski ME (1999) High resolution imaging of normal and osteoarthritic cartilage with optical coherence tomography. J Rheumatol 26(3):627–635

32. Hungerford DS, Barry M (1979) Biomechanics of the patellofemoral joint. Clin Orthop Relat Res 144:9–15

33. Insall J, Falvo KA, Wise DW (1976) Chondromalacia patellae: a prospective study. J Bone Jt Surg Am Vol 58-A(1):1–8

34. Jackson RW, Abe I (1972) The role of arthroscopy in the management of disorders of the knee: an analysis of 200 consecutive examinations. J Bone Jt Surg Br Vol 54-B(2):310–322

35. Jiang CC, Liu YJ, Yip KM, Wu E (1993) Physiological patellofemoral crepitus in knee joint disorders. Bull Hosp Jt Dis 53(4):22–26

36. Jiang CC, Lee JH, Yuan TT (2000) Vibration arthrometry in the patients with failed total knee replacement. IEEE Trans Biomed Eng 47(2):218–227

37. Kellgren JH, Lawrence JS (1957) Radiological assessment of osteo-arthrosis. Ann Rheum Dis 16:494–501

38. Kernohan WG, Beverland DE, McCoy GF, Hamilton A, Watson P, Mollan RAB (1990) Vibration arthrometry. Acta Orthop Scand 61(1):70–79

39. Kernohan WG, Barr DA, McCoy GF, Mollan RAB (1991) Vibration arthrometry in assessment of knee disorders: the problem of angular velocity. J Biomed Eng 13:35–38

40. Kim KS, Seo JH, Kang JU, Song CG (2009) An enhanced algorithm for knee joint sound classification using feature extraction based on time-frequency analysis. Comput Methods Programs Biomed 94(2):198–206

41. Kiviranta P, Lammentausta E, Toyras J, Kiviranta I, Jurvelin JS (2008) Indentation diagnostics of cartilage degeneration. Osteoarthr Cartil 16(7):796–804

42. Krishnan S, Rangayyan RM (2000) Automatic de-noising of knee-joint vibration signals using adaptive time-frequency representations. Med Biol Eng Comput 38(8):2–8

43. Krishnan S, Rangayyan RM, Bell GD, Frank CB, Ladly KO (1997) Adaptive filtering, modelling, and classification of knee joint vibroarthrographic signals for non-invasive diagnosis of articular cartilage pathology. Med Biol Eng Comput 35(6):677–684

44. Krishnan S, Rangayyan RM, Bell GD, Frank CB (2000) Adaptive time-frequency analysis of knee joint vibroarthrographic signals for noninvasive screening of articular cartilage pathology. IEEE Trans Biomed Eng 47(6):773–783

45. Krishnan S, Rangayyan RM, Bell GD, Frank CB (2001) Auditory display of knee-joint vibration signals. J Acoust Soc Am 110(6):3292–3304

46. Lee JH, Jiang CC, Yuan TT (2000) Vibration arthrometry in patients with knee joint disorders. IEEE Trans Biomed Eng 47(8):1131–1133
47. Li LP, Herzog W (2006) Arthroscopic evaluation of cartilage degeneration using indentation testing–influence of indenter geometry. Clin Biomech 21(4):420–426
48. Li X, Martin S, Pitris C, Ghanta R, Stamper DL, Harman M, Fujimoto JG, Brezinski ME (2005) High-resolution optical coherence tomographic imaging of osteoarthritic cartilage during open knee surgery. Arthritis Res Ther 7(2):R318–R323
49. Lund F, Nilsson BE (1980) Arthroscopy of the patello-femoral joint. Acta Orthop Scand 51:297–302
50. Manaster BJ, Crim J, Rosenberg ZS (2007) Diagnostic and surgical imaging anatomy: knee, ankle, foot. Lippincott Williams and Wilkins, Philadelphia
51. Mankin HJ (1982) The response of articular-cartilage to mechanical injury. J Bone Jt Surg Am Vol 64-A(3):462–466
52. McCoy GF, McCrea JD, Beverland DE, Kernohan WG, Mollan RAB (1987) Vibration arthrography as a diagnostic aid in diseases of the knee: a preliminary report. J Bone Jt Surg Br Vol 69-B(2):288–293
53. Metcalf RW (1984) Arthroscopic knee surgery. Adv Surg 17:197–240
54. Mollan RAB, McCullagh GC, Wilson RI (1982) A critical appraisal of auscultation of human joints. Clin Orthop Relat Res 170:231–237
55. Mollan RAB, Kernohan WG, Watters PH (1983) Artefact encountered by the vibration detection system. J Biomech 16(3):193–199
56. Moller I, Dong D, Naredo E, Filippucci E, Carrasco I, Moragues C, Iagnocco A (2008) Ultrasound in the study and monitoring of osteoarthritis. Osteoarthr Cartil 16(Suppl 3):S4–S7
57. Moore KL, Dalley AF (2005) Clinically oriented anatomy, 5th edn. Lippincott Williams and Wilkins, Philadelphia
58. Moussavi ZMK, Rangayyan RM, Bell GD, Frank CB, Ladly KO, Zhang YT (1996) Screening of vibroarthrographic signals via adaptive segmentation and linear prediction modeling. IEEE Trans Biomed Eng 43(1):15–23
59. Mu T, Nandi AK, Rangayyan RM (2008) Screening of knee-joint vibroarthrographic signals using the strict 2-surface proximal classifier and genetic algorithm. Comput Biol Med 38(10):1103–1111
60. Noyes FR, Stabler CL (1989) A system for grading articular cartilage lesions at arthroscopy. Am J Sports Med 17(4):505–513
61. Outerbridge RE, Dunlop JA (1975) The problem of chondromalacia patellae. Clin Orthop Relat Res 110:177–196
62. Peylan A (1953) Direct auscultation of the joints (preliminary clinical observations). Rheumatism 9:77–81
63. Rabin EL, Ehrlich MG, Cherrack R, Abermathy P, Paul IL, Rose RM (1978) Effect of repetitive impulsive loading on the knee joints of rabbits. Clin Orthop 131:288–293
64. Rangayyan RM (2002) Biomedical signal analysis: a case-study approach. IEEE/Wiley, New York
65. Rangayyan RM, Wu YF (2008) Screening of knee-joint vibroarthrographic signals using statistical parameters and radial basis functions. Med Biol Eng Comput 46(3):223–232
66. Rangayyan RM, Wu Y (2009) Analysis of vibroarthrographic signals with features related to signal variability and radial-basis functions. Ann Biomed Eng 37(1):156–163
67. Rangayyan RM, Wu Y (2010) Screening of knee-joint vibroarthrographic signals using probability density functions estimated with Parzen windows. Biomed Signal Process Control 5(1):53–58
68. Rangayyan RM, Krishnan S, Bell GD, Frank CB, Ladly KO (1997) Parametric representation and screening of knee joint vibroarthrographic signals. IEEE Trans Biomed Eng 44(11): 1068–1074
69. Rangayyan RM, Oloumi F, Wu Y, Cai S (2013) Fractal analysis of knee-joint vibroarthrographic signals via power spectral analysis. Biomed Signal Process Control 8(1):26–29
70. Rashidifard C, Vercollone C, Martin S, Liu B, Brezinski ME (2013) The application of optical coherence tomography in musculoskeletal disease. Arthritis 2013:563268

71. Reddy NP, Rothschild BM, Mandal M, Gupta V, Suryanarayanan S (1995) Noninvasive acceleration measurements to characterize knee arthritis and chondromalacia. Ann Biomed Eng 23(1):78–84
72. Reddy NP, Rothschild BM, Verrall E, Joshi A (2001) Noninvasive measurement of acceleration at the knee joint in patients with rheumatoid arthritis and spondyloarthropathy of the knee. Ann Biomed Eng 29(12):1106–1111
73. Shen YP, Rangayyan RM, Bell GD, Frank CB, Zhang YT, Ladly KO (1995) Localization of knee joint cartilage pathology by multichannel vibroarthrography. Med Eng Phys 17(8):583–594
74. Small NC (1990) Complications in arthroscopic meniscal surgery. Clin Sports Med 9(3):609–617
75. Smillie IS (1978) Injuries of the knee joint, 5th edn. Churchill Livingstone, Edinburgh
76. Sonin AH, Pensy RA, Mulligan ME, Hatem S (2002) Grading articular cartilage of the knee using fast spin-echo proton density-weighted MR imaging without fat suppression. Am J Roentgenol 179(5):1159–1166
77. Starkey C, Ryan J (2002) Evaluation of orthopedic and athletic injuries, 2nd edn. F. A. Davis Company, Philadelphia
78. Steindler A (1937) Auscultation of joints. J Bone Jt Surg 19(1):121–136
79. Symmons D, Mathers C, Pfleger B (15-8-2006 edition, 2006) The global burden of osteoarthritis in the year 2000: GBD 2000 working paper draft. World Health Organization, Geneva
80. Tanaka N, Hoshiyama M (2012) Vibroarthrography in patients with knee arthropathy. J Back Musculoskelet Rehabil 25(2):117–122
81. Tavathia S, Rangayyan RM, Frank CB, Bell GD, Ladly KO, Zhang YT (1992) Analysis of knee vibration signals using linear prediction. IEEE Trans Biomed Eng 39(9):959–970
82. Tortora GJ (2004) Principles of human anatomy, 10th edn. Wiley, New York
83. Umapathy K, Krishnan S (2006) Modified local discriminant bases algorithm and its application in analysis of human knee joint vibration signals. IEEE Trans Biomed Eng 53(3):517–523
84. van Leersum M, Schweitzer ME, Gannon F, Finkel G, Vinitski S, Mitchell DG (1996) Chondromalacia patellae: an in vitro study. Comparison of MR criteria with histologic and macroscopic findings. Skelet Radiol 25(8):727–732
85. Vignon E, Conrozier T, Piperno M, Richard S, Carrillon Y, Fantino O (1999) Radiographic assessment of hip and knee osteoarthritis. Recommendations: recommended guidelines. Osteoarthr Cartil 7(4):434–436
86. Vigorita VJ (1999) Orthopaedic pathology. Lippincott Williams and Wilkins, Philadelphia
87. Walters CF (1929) The value of joint auscultation. Lancet 1:920–921
88. Wiles P, Andrews PS, Bremner RA (1960) Chondromalacia of the patella. J Bone Jt Surg Br Vol 42-B(1):65–70
89. Wu Y, Krishnan S (2011) Combining least-squares support vector machines for classification of biomedical signals: a case study with knee-joint vibroarthrographic signals. J Exp Theor Artif Intell 23(1):63–77
90. Wu Y, Krishnan S, Rangayyan RM (2010) Computer-aided diagnosis of knee-joint disorders via vibroarthrographic signal analysis: a review. Crit Rev Biomed Eng 38(2):201–224
91. Wu Y, Cai S, Yang S, Zheng F, Xiang N (2013) Classification of knee joint vibration signals using bivariate feature distribution estimation and maximal posterior probability decision criterion. Entropy 15(4):1375–1387
92. Wu Y, Yang S, Zheng F, Cai S, Lu M, Wu M (2014) Removal of artifacts in knee joint vibroarthrographic signals using ensemble empirical mode decomposition and detrended fluctuation analysis. Physiol Meas 35(3):429–439
93. Yang S, Cai S, Zheng F, Wu Y, Liu K, Wu M, Zou Q, Chen J (2014) Representation of fluctuation features in pathological knee joint vibroarthrographic signals using kernel density modeling method. Med Eng Phys 36(10):1305–1311

Chapter 2
Signal Acquisition and Preprocessing

Abstract This chapter describes the detailed settings of the knee joint vibroarthrographic signal acquisition system. The text also presents a cascade moving average filter method to estimate the baseline wander in the raw signal, along with the combination of the ensemble empirical mode decomposition and detrended fluctuation analysis algorithms to remove the random noise. The filtering techniques for reduction of muscle contraction interference are also reviewed in the chapter.

2.1 Signal Analysis Procedures

The common flowchart of VAG signal analysis procedures is shown in Fig. 2.1. The data acquisition system collects the raw time series and conditions the signal with bandpass filters and amplifiers. The task of the signal preprocessing procedure is to remove the artifacts in the raw signal. Such artifacts mainly include baseline wander, random noise, and periodical power-line interference. With the artifact-free signal, several computational methods can then be employed to study the signal in the time scale or time-frequency domain. Advanced approaches can also be applied to characterize the fractal and statistical properties of the VAG signal. The distinct features extracted from the signal provide the particular information about the signal variability and complexity in waveform shifting, frequency range, or statistics [16–18]. The feature computing procedure mainly focuses on combining and refining the most informative feature sets, by using feature selection or mapping techniques [20]. Finally, the pattern analysis tools can be utilized to distinguish the pathological signals recorded from symptomatic patients and the normal signals recorded from healthy subjects [3, 28, 34].

2.2 Signal Acquisition

As shown in Fig. 2.2, VAG signals can be recorded with one or more accelerometers [9, 21, 22] or an electro-stethoscope [8]. The sensor can be taped to the subject's patella [21, 22, 24], middle of the patella [9, 24, 38], lateral condyle of the tibia

© The Author(s) 2015
Y. Wu, *Knee Joint Vibroarthrographic Signal Processing and Analysis,*
SpringerBriefs in Bioengineering, DOI 10.1007/978-3-662-44284-5_2

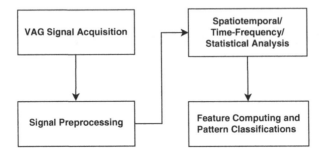

Fig. 2.1 Diagram of knee joint VAG signal analysis methodology

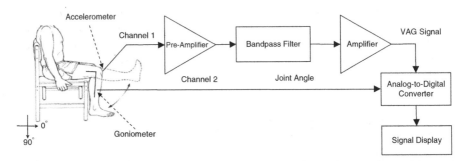

Fig. 2.2 Knee joint vibroarthrographic (*VAG*) data acquisition setup. Channel 1 records the VAG signal at the middle position of patella; channel 2 records goniometer voltage (angle) information

[24, 25, 38], medial condyle of the tibia [8, 24], or tibial tuberosity [24, 38], by using two-sided adhesive tapes. The subjects are commonly asked to bend the leg at the knee joint (reducing the angle between the shank and thigh), and straighten the leg until the full knee extension. The accelerometer sensor can measure the acceleration and deceleration amplitude of the knee joint in the course of flexion or extension. In addition to the accelerometer or stethoscope sensor, a VAG signal acquisition system may also consist of an electro-goniometer in order to measure the bending angle of the leg during the knee flexion or extension. Before the signal recording, it is necessary to appropriately configure the supporting devices and software, which commonly contain anti-aliasing bandpass filters, amplifiers, analog-to-digital converter, graphic signal display, and signal condition toolkits.

This book presents the VAG signal acquisition system and the experimental protocol developed by the research group of Rangayyan [10, 12, 19, 24, 36], as a paradigm. A miniature accelerometer (Model 3115A, Dytran Instruments, Inc., Chatsworth, CA, USA) was adhered to the middle of the patella. The subjects were requested to sit on a rigid chair with the legs both freely suspended in air. During the signal recording procedure, each subject should voluntarily swing the shank tested over an angle range from 135° to 0° (extension movement), and back to 135° (flexion movement) in the duration of 4 s [19] (associated with an approximate angular velocity of 67° per second).

The raw time series was collected by an instrumentation recorder (Model 3968A, Hewlett Packard, San Diego, CA, USA) with a sampling rate of 2 kHz. Then, the acceleration signal was conditioned by a bandpass filter with a bandwidth of 10 Hz– 1 kHz to prevent aliasing effects, and amplified by isolation pre-amplifiers (Model 11-5407-58, Gould Instrument Systems, Inc., Cleveland, OH, USA) and universal amplifiers (Model 13-4615-18, Gould Instrument Systems, Inc., Cleveland, OH, USA). The signal was digitized with a resolution of 12 bit per sample by using a data acquisition board (AT-MIO-16L, National Instruments, Austin, TX, USA) and the LabVIEW software (National Instruments, Austin, TX, USA).

Auscultation of the knee joint using a stethoscope was also performed to provide a qualitative description of sound intensity, along with the corresponding relationship to the angle of knee joint. For the subjects who underwent arthroscopic surgery, the lesion locations observed were used to estimate the joint angles at which the appeared articular surfaces would come into contact and affect the corresponding VAG signal segments.

2.3 Signal Preprocessing

In clinical application, it is essential to record high-quality VAG signals for computer-aided diagnostic analysis of knee joint pathology [32]. However, recording of the knee joint VAG signals with the sensor on the contact surface of the subject's patella is susceptible to several different types of artifacts, including electromyogram, random noise, ambient interference, and baseline wander [2, 33]. The artifact of electromyogram is commonly induced by concurrent muscular contractions during the knee flexion or extension motion. Random noise due to the thermal effect in the ambient cables and amplifiers is inevitable in the signal acquisition procedure. Since the mechanism of random noise is complex and random, the range of signal-to-noise ratio of VAG signals cannot be determined a priori [32]. The major environmental interference is caused by 50 or 60 Hz power-supply lines and radio-frequency emissions from medical devices. However, the signal acquisition system driven by direct-current battery power supply is free of the periodical power-line interference. Sometimes, patients with knee joint disorders may tremble the legs due to skin friction or the painful reaction when they bending the leg in a vibration arthrometry examination, which would cause the baseline wander in the raw signal.

2.3.1 Removal of Baseline Wander

In order to remove the baseline wander in the VAG record, we may use a cascade moving average filter to estimate the such a artifact and then subtract it from the raw signal [2]. The moving average filter is a type of finite impulse response (FIR) filter

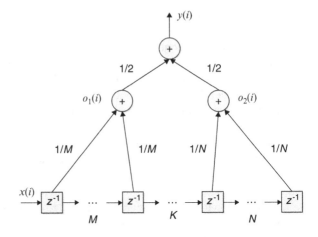

Fig. 2.3 The hierarchical structure of the cascade moving average filter

that is frequently used for time series analysis. In the filtering procedure, temporal statistics are computed using a few samples of the signal along the time axis, and the samples in a temporal moving window are averaged to produce the output at various points of time [15]. Different from the conventional design of a moving average filter, the cascade moving average filter consists of a hierarchical structure that combines two-layer moving average operators, as shown in Fig. 2.3. The first layer of the cascade filter includes a M-order and a N-order successive moving average operators. The K inputs in the tail end of the M-order operator overlap with the beginning inputs of the N-order operator. The output of the M-order operator $o_1(i)$ is written as

$$o_1(i) = \frac{1}{M} [x(i-1) + \cdots + x(i-M)]$$

$$= \frac{1}{M} \sum_{m=1}^{M} x(i-m), \tag{2.1}$$

and the output of the following N-order operator $o_2(i)$ can be expressed as

$$o_2(i) = \frac{1}{N} [x(i-M+K) + \cdots + x(i-M+K-N)]$$

$$= \frac{1}{N} \sum_{n=1}^{N} x(i-M+K-n). \tag{2.2}$$

The second layer of the moving average filter is designed to smooth the piecewise linear trends obtained from the outputs of two moving average operators in the first layer. The final output of the cascade moving average filter is given by

$$y(i) = [o_1(i) + o_2(i)]/2$$

$$= \frac{1}{2M} \sum_{m=1}^{M} x(i - m) + \frac{1}{2N} \sum_{n=1}^{N} x(i - M + K - n). \qquad (2.3)$$

By applying the z-transform, we may compute the transfer function $H(z)$ of the cascade moving average filter as

$$H(z) = \frac{Y(z)}{X(z)} = \frac{1}{2M} \left(z^{-1} + \cdots + z^{-M} \right) + \frac{1}{2N} \left(z^{-M+K-1} + \cdots + z^{-M+K-N} \right), \qquad (2.4)$$

where $X(z)$ and $Y(z)$ are the z-transform of the filter input $x(i)$ and output $y(i)$, respectively.

To estimate the baseline wander in the VAG signal, the two moving average operators in the first layer of the hierarchical model can be configured with the equal orders, i.e., $M = 20$ and $N = 20$, respectively. The reason for such a filter design is due to the symmetry of the leg swinging angles ($135° \rightarrow 0° \rightarrow 135°$) in the signal acquisition experiment. The number of the overlapping inputs of the moving average operators is set to be $K = 5$. The frequency response of the cascade moving average filter is shown in Fig. 2.4.

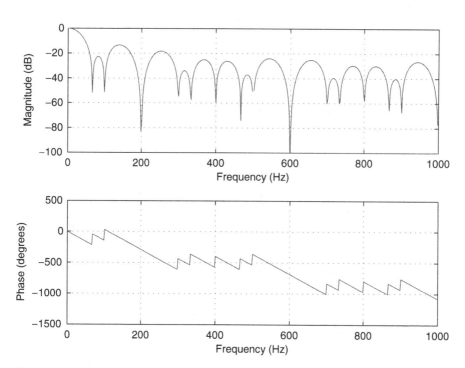

Fig. 2.4 The frequency response of the cascade moving average filter for detrending the baseline wander in knee joint vibroarthrographic signal

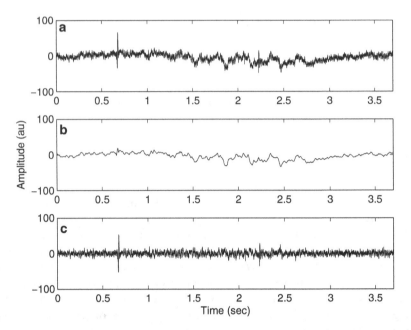

Fig. 2.5 Subfigures from top to bottom: (**a**) the raw knee joint vibroarthrographic signal recorded from a healthy subject, (**b**) the baseline wander estimated by the cascade moving average filter, and (**c**) the baseline-wander-free signal of the filter output

The results of baseline wander removal in the VAG signals for a healthy subject and a patient (33-year-old male) with Grade II-III chondromalacia patellae are plotted in Figs. 2.5 and 2.6, respectively. It is noted that the normal VAG signal in Fig. 2.5a is contaminated with a few random noise, but the signal variation is relatively small in amplitude. The abnormal VAG signal in Fig. 2.6a dramatically fluctuates from 0.8 to 1.25 s, and later from 1.8 to 2.3 s, which corresponds to the pathological joint surface at the angle range from 30° to 110°. It can be observed from Fig. 2.5b that the baseline wander in the normal signal exhibits higher degree of regularity in the waveform than that in the pathological signal shown in Fig. 2.6b. The baseline wander estimated in Fig. 2.6b is caused due to the uncomfortable trembling of the leg in the course of knee extension and flexion through the degenerative joint surface. It is noted from Figs. 2.5c and 2.6c that the drifts have been effectively eliminated by the cascade moving average filter, and the baselines of the filtered VAG signals are placed back to the isoelectric line (the zero level).

2.3.2 Removal of Random Noise

The noise in the form of random fluctuations around the isoelectric line is a common type of artifacts in biomedical signals [11, 29, 31, 33]. The random noise could

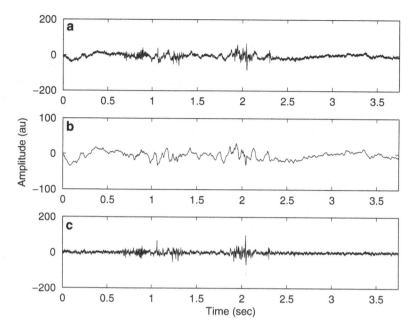

Fig. 2.6 Subfigures from top to bottom: (**a**) the raw knee joint vibroarthrographic signal recorded from a patient (male, age: 33 years old) with Grade II-III chondromalacia patellae, (**b**) the baseline wander estimated by the cascade moving average filter, and (**c**) the baseline-wander-free signal output by the cascade moving average filter

be generated due to the unavoidable thermal effect or semiconductor defects of medical instruments [30]. In this section, we introduce an effective method that combines the ensemble empirical mode decomposition and detrended fluctuation analysis algorithms to remove random noise in the VAG signal [35]. The EEMD first divides the raw VAG signal into several intrinsic mode functions (IMFs) in the successive decomposition processes. The DFA algorithm is then applied to identify the inherent correlation property of each IMF. Finally, the IMFs that contain the dominant artifacts of random noise and monotonic baseline residue can be removed in the reconstructed artifact-reduced signal.

2.3.2.1 Ensemble Empirical Mode Decomposition

The empirical mode decomposition (EMD) was introduced by Huang et al. [4] as a popular technique for nonlinear and nonstationary signal analysis. The EMD method works by sifting a given signal into a set of intrinsic mode functions (IMFs) that represent the fast and slow oscillations in the signal [5]. Although this rationale shares much with the wavelet analysis philosophy, the IMFs with slow oscillations are not defined through any prescribed filtering operation [23]. For each IMF, the local maxima are all positive and the local minima are all negative [33].

The envelops of the IMFs defined in the sifting operator are zero-crossing and symmetrical. For a signal that is composed of two or more spectral components, the EMD method has the capability to separate these components with different amplitude levels in the decomposed IMFs, as confirmed in the previous work of Rilling and Flandrin [23]. However, the effectiveness of the EMD method is limited by the mode mixing effect [6]. Mode mixing is a phenomenon that the oscillations with disparate time scales are preserved in one IMF, or that the oscillations with the same time scale are sifted into different IMFs.

Recently, Wu and Huang [27] proposed a noise-assisted EMD algorithm, called ensemble empirical mode decomposition (EEMD), to overcome the mode mixing obstacle. The EEMD adds different series of white noise into the signal in several trials [35]. The added white noise plays a crucial role in the decomposition process, because it provides uniformly distributed references of different scales [26]. In each trial, the added noise is different, such that the decomposed IMFs have no correlation with the corresponding IMFs from one trial to another. If the number of trials is sufficient, the added noise can be canceled out by ensemble averaging of the corresponding IMFs obtained in the different trials. The details of the EEMD process are described as follows [27].

1. In the nth trial, a white noise time series $u_n(t)$ is added to a given signal $x(t)$, in order to attain a new time series $y_n(t) = x(t) + u_n(t), n = 1, 2, \ldots, N$, where N denotes the number of ensemble.
2. The noise-contaminated signal $y_n(t)$ is decomposed into a set of IMFs using the original EMD method [4], that is

$$y_n(t) = \sum_{j=1}^{i} c_j^n + r_i^n, \tag{2.5}$$

where i denotes the total number of the IMFs in each decomposition, c_j^n is the jth IMF, and r_i^n represents the residue of $y_n(t)$ in the nth trial. To ensure that the number of IMFs in each decomposition to be equal, we may assign a fixed siftings number of 10, so as to produce the IMF in each VAG signal decomposition process.
3. The above two steps are repeated for N trials, with different white noise series $u_n(t)$ added in each trial.
4. The corresponding jth IMFs obtained in the total N trials are averaged, that is

$$c_j^{ave} = \frac{1}{N} \sum_{n=1}^{N} c_j^n, \tag{2.6}$$

where c_j^{ave} is the final IMF of the EEMD.

The effectiveness of the EEMD method depends on the appropriate setting of the ensemble number and the amplitude of added white noise. Wu and Huang [27] suggested that the number of ensemble (N) and the amplitude of added noise (A) should satisfy the following rule:

$$\varepsilon = \frac{A}{\sqrt{N}}, \tag{2.7}$$

where ε represents the final standard deviation of error, which indicates the difference between the original data and the sum of the IMFs produced by the EEMD method. The ratio of the standard deviation of the added noise and that of the raw VAG signal could be 0.2. And the number of ensemble could be fixed at $N = 100$ to average the corresponding IMFs obtained in the total 100 trials of the EEMD.

Figure 2.7 shows the IMFs decomposed by the EEMD method from the VAG signal of a patient with anterior cruciate ligament (ACL) and chondromalacia in the knee. The EEMD provided the C1–C11 IMFs in the successive decomposition iterations, and remained the monotonic trend as the final residue. It is visualized in Fig. 2.7 that different IMFs exhibit the components of the raw signal with different levels of fluctuations. The first three IMFs (C1–C3) are composed of most of the fast (high-frequency) oscillations in the raw VAG signal. The IMFs decomposed at the higher levels (C4–C11), on the other hand, consist of more slow (low-frequency) oscillations. The distinct morphological characteristics associated with the pathological conditions of ACL (from 0.9 to 1.1 s and from 3.7 to 4 s) and chondromalacia (from 1.4 to 1.9 s) can be observed in the C4–C6 IMFs in Fig. 2.7.

2.3.2.2 Fractal Scaling Index

With the IMFs decomposed by the EEMD method, the next task is to identify whether an IMF contains the dominant artifacts in the knee joint VAG signal. In most cases, the artifacts and the signal components possess different correlation properties (for example, anti-correlated or long-range correlated). The detrended fluctuation analysis (DFA) algorithm can be applied to study such correlation properties of each IMF [35]. It is very popular for the detection of nonstationary time series that exhibit long-range correlation properties [1]. The DFA algorithm computes the fractal scaling index parameter that describes the subtle fluctuations associated with intrinsic correlations of the dynamics in the signal. The fractal scaling index (α) is often used to measure the statistical self-affinity of a signal [13, 14].

Given an L-length decomposed IMF $c_j^{ave}(l)$ with the mean value of w_j, the integrated IMF time series $s(m)$ is defined by

$$s(m) = \sum_{l=1}^{m} \left[c_j^{ave}(l) - w_j \right]. \tag{2.8}$$

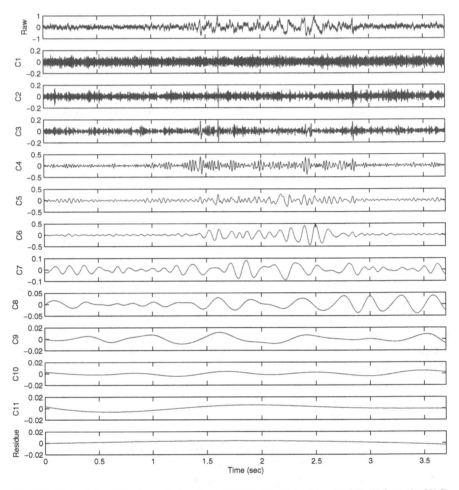

Fig. 2.7 Plots of the intrinsic mode functions (IMFs) decomposed by the EEMD from the VAG signal of a patient with anterior cruciate ligament and chondromalacia. From top to bottom: the raw signal, the corresponding IMFs (C1–C11), and the monotonic trend (Residue)

The integrated time series $s(m)$ is then divided into several window segments of equal size k, and a least-squares line (i.e., the local linear trend), denoted as $s_k(m)$, that fits the window samples. The local detrended fluctuation is then computed by subtracting the local linear trend $s_k(m)$ from the integrated time series $s(m)$ in each window segment. The averaged fluctuation $F(k)$ is computed with the local detrended fluctuations in the root-mean-square sense as

$$F(k) = \left[\frac{1}{L} \sum_{m=1}^{L} [s(m) - s_k(m)]^2 \right]^{\frac{1}{2}}. \tag{2.9}$$

For the VAG signal sampled at 2 kHz, the averaged fluctuation computation could be iteratively performed over the time scales defined by the window sizes in the range of from 10 to 250, with an increment of 20, for each decomposed IMF. The function relating the averaged fluctuation $F(k)$ to the window size k is usually plotted with a double logarithmic graph. The fractal scaling index (α) is defined as the slope of the linear relationship between $\log_{10} F(k)$ and $\log_{10} k$, which is expressed by a power law as $F(k) \sim k^{\alpha}$ [14]. In the case of $0.5 < \alpha < 1$, the integrated and detrended time series possess persistent long-range power-law correlations, whereas $0 < \alpha < 0.5$ indicates an anti-correlated property of the time series [7]. Typically, the fractal scaling index $\alpha = 0.5$ indicates the integrated and detrended time series is considered as white noise [13]. For the pink noise ($1/f$ noise) and Brown noise, the fractal scaling index values of the integrated and detrended time series are $\alpha = 1$ and $\alpha = 1.5$, respectively [13].

To identify the artifact components in the VAG signal, the DFA algorithm is implemented to compute the fractal scaling index (α) value for each IMF. The double-logarithmic relationships between the averaged fluctuation and the window size for the C1, C6, and C8 IMFs are displayed in Fig. 2.8. It is clear that these three IMFs possess different α values, i.e., the slope of the linear fitting in the root-mean-square sense. The fractal scaling index value of the C1 IMF is equal to 0.14, which

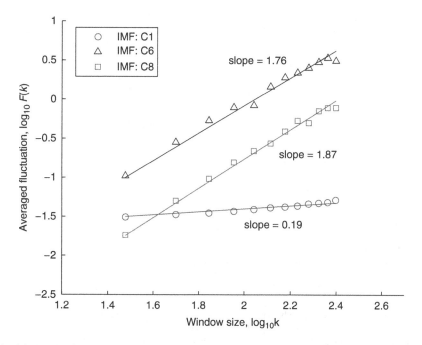

Fig. 2.8 Double logarithmic plots of the linear relationship between averaged fluctuation $F(k)$ and the window size k, for the IMFs C1, C6, and C8, decomposed from the VAG signal of a patient with anterior cruciate ligament and chondromalacia

indicates that such an IMF contains plenty of anti-correlated components. The α values of the C6 and C8 IMFs are larger than 1.5, which implies that both of these IMFs are with long-range power-law correlations. The C6 IMF ($\alpha = 1.6$) involves less long-range correlated components than the C8 IMF ($\alpha = 1.86$), because the C6 IMFs contains more fast oscillations of the VAG signal. Since the random noise are not long-range correlated, the VAG signal can be reconstructed with the long-range correlated IMFs ($\alpha > 0.5$), such that the IMFs with anti-correlations ($0 < \alpha < 0.5$) and the final monotonic residue (baseline wander) are considered as artifacts. A comparison of the raw VAG signal and the reconstructed artifact-reduced signal is shown in Fig. 2.9. It is clear that the removed artifacts in Fig. 2.9b contains a larger number of fast oscillations, and the morphological segments associated with the pathological conditions are not distorted in the artifact-free VAG signal in Fig. 2.9c. It is also worth noting that there still exist some components with rapidly variations in the reconstructed VAG signal in Fig. 2.9c. These long-range correlated components are the mechanomyographic and vibromyographic responses of the superficial muscles contracted in the duration of knee flexion and extension in the signal acquisition procedure.

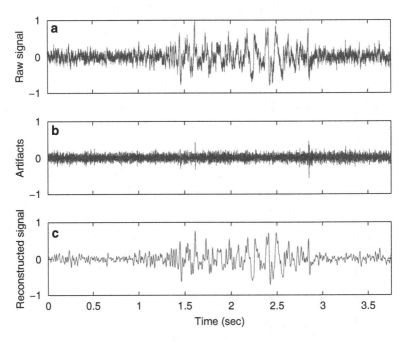

Fig. 2.9 Subfigures from top to bottom: (**a**) the raw knee joint vibroarthrographic signal a patient with anterior cruciate ligament and chondromalacia, (**b**) the noise components decomposed by the ensemble empirical mode decomposition method, and (**c**) the reconstructed artifact-free signal

2.3.3 Reduction of Muscle Contraction Interference

Muscle contraction interference (MCI) is another type of dominant artifacts that may obscure the VAG signal analysis. MCI involves the effects of vibromyogram (VMG) associated with contraction of skeletal muscles [37, 39]. The VMG signal, also known as the muscle sound, is the acoustic manifestation of the mechanical activity of muscle fibers, and can be detected with accelerometers placed on the skin surface over an active muscle. Zhang et al. [37] compared simultaneous recordings of VMG and electromygram (EMG) generated by skeletal muscles during voluntary isometric and isotonic contractions. Their results suggested that the VMG and EMG signals are equally sensitive to muscle contraction levels at various joint angles, and that the frequency and intensity of the VMG signal vary in direct proportion to the muscular contraction level. To reduce the MCI, Zhang et al. [39] applied a two-stage least-mean-squares (LMS) adaptive filter. The first stage was used to remove the measurement noise in the accelerometers and associated amplifiers, and the second stage was designed to cancel the muscle signal. The step size of the LMS adaptive filter was optimized by using a root-mean-squared-error-based gradient noise (or misadjustment) factor and a time-varying estimate of the input signal power [36]. The MCI reference was recorded with an accelerometer placed on the skin at the distal rectus femoris position using two-sided adhesive tapes. Krishnan et al. [10] improved the adaptive MCI cancellation technique with a 6th-order recursive least-squares (RLS) adaptive filter with the forgetting factor fixed at 0.98. The RLS adaptive filter provided two major advantages over the LMS adaptive filter. First, the convergence of the RLS algorithm was faster than that of the LMS algorithm. Second, the parameter (forgetting factor) of the RLS adaptive filter could be fixed, whereas the step size of the LMS filter had to be optimized with reference to input signal power, which varies with time spans. The results of the experiments of Krishnan et al. [10] indicated that MCI filtering was not an essential preprocessing step before feature extraction, and that the adaptive MCI cancellation step could make the results of VAG signal classification even worse. Based on such a conclusion, several subsequent studies related to VAG signal analysis [9, 16–18, 20] did not include the step of MCI reduction.

References

1. Bak P, Tang C, Wiesenfeld K (1987) Self-organized criticality: an explanation of the $1/f$ noise. Phys Rev Lett 59:381–384
2. Cai S, Wu Y, Xiang N, Zhong Z, He J, Shi L, Xu F (2012) Detrending knee joint vibration signals with a cascade moving average filter. In: Proceedings of the 34th annual international conference of IEEE engineering in medicine and biology society, San Diego, pp 4357–4360
3. Cai S, Yang S, Zheng F, Lu M, Wu Y, Krishnan S (2013) Knee joint vibration signal analysis with matching pursuit decomposition and dynamic weighted classifier fusion. Comput Math Methods Med 2013:Article ID 904267

4. Huang NE, Shen Z, Long SR, Wu MC, Shih HH, Zheng Q, Yen NC, Tung CC, Liu HH (1998) The empirical mode decomposition and the Hilbert spectrum for nonlinear and non-stationary time series analysis. Proc R Soc Lond A 454:903–995

5. Huang NE, Shen Z, Long SR (1999) A new view of nonlinear water waves: the Hilbert spectrum. Annu Rev Fluid Mech 31(1):417–457

6. Huang NE, Wu MLC, Long SR, Shen SSP, Qu W, Gloersen P, Fan KL (2003) A confidence limit for the empirical mode decomposition and Hilbert spectral analysis. Proc R Soc Lond Ser A: Math, Phys Eng Sci 459(2037):2317–2345

7. Kantelhardt JW, Koscielny-Bunde E, Rego HH, Havlin S, Bunde A (2001) Detecting long-range correlations with detrended fluctuation analysis. Physica A 295(3):441–454

8. Kim KS, Seo JH, Kang JU, Song CG (2009) An enhanced algorithm for knee joint sound classification using feature extraction based on time-frequency analysis. Comput Methods Programs Biomed 94(2):198–206

9. Krishnan S, Rangayyan RM (2000) Automatic de-noising of knee-joint vibration signals using adaptive time-frequency representations. Med Biol Eng Comput 38(8):2–8

10. Krishnan S, Rangayyan RM, Bell GD, Frank CB, Ladly KO (1997) Adaptive filtering, modelling, and classification of knee joint vibroarthrographic signals for non-invasive diagnosis of articular cartilage pathology. Med Biol Eng Comput 35(6):677–684

11. Lu M, Cai S, Zheng F, Yang S, Xiang N, Wu Y (2012) Adaptive noise removal of knee joint vibration signals using a signal power error minimization method. In: Proceedings of the 7th international conference on computing and convergence technology, Seoul, pp 1193–1196

12. Moussavi ZMK, Rangayyan RM, Bell GD, Frank CB, Ladly KO, Zhang YT (1996) Screening of vibroarthrographic signals via adaptive segmentation and linear prediction modeling. IEEE Trans Biomed Eng 43(1):15–23

13. Peng CK, Buldyrev SV, Goldberger AL, Havlin S, Sciortino F, Simons M, Stanley HE (1992) Long-range correlations in nucleotide sequences. Nature 356:168–170

14. Peng CK, Havlin S, Stanley HE, Goldberger AL (1995) Quantification of scaling exponents and crossover phenomena in nonstationary heartbeat time series. Chaos 5(1):82–87

15. Rangayyan RM (2002) Biomedical signal analysis: a case-study approach. IEEE/Wiley, New York

16. Rangayyan RM, Wu YF (2008) Screening of knee-joint vibroarthrographic signals using statistical parameters and radial basis functions. Med Biol Eng Comput 46(3):223–232

17. Rangayyan RM, Wu Y (2009) Analysis of vibroarthrographic signals with features related to signal variability and radial-basis functions. Ann Biomed Eng 37(1):156–163

18. Rangayyan RM, Wu Y (2010) Screening of knee-joint vibroarthrographic signals using probability density functions estimated with Parzen windows. Biomed Signal Process Control 5(1):53–58

19. Rangayyan RM, Krishnan S, Bell GD, Frank CB, Ladly KO (1997) Parametric representation and screening of knee joint vibroarthrographic signals. IEEE Trans Biomed Eng 44(11): 1068–1074

20. Rangayyan RM, Oloumi F, Wu Y, Cai S (2013) Fractal analysis of knee-joint vibroarthrographic signals via power spectral analysis. Biomed Signal Process Control 8(1):26–29

21. Reddy NP, Rothschild BM, Mandal M, Gupta V, Suryanarayanan S (1995) Noninvasive acceleration measurements to characterize knee arthritis and chondromalacia. Ann Biomed Eng 23(1):78–84

22. Reddy NP, Rothschild BM, Verrall E, Joshi A (2001) Noninvasive measurement of acceleration at the knee joint in patients with rheumatoid arthritis and spondyloarthropathy of the knee. Ann Biomed Eng 29(12):1106–1111

23. Rilling G, Flandrin P (2008) One or two frequencies? The empirical mode decomposition answers. IEEE Trans Signal Process 56(1):85–95

24. Shen YP, Rangayyan RM, Bell GD, Frank CB, Zhang YT, Ladly KO (1995) Localization of knee joint cartilage pathology by multichannel vibroarthrography. Med Eng Phys 17(8): 583–594

25. Tanaka N, Hoshiyama M (2012) Vibroarthrography in patients with knee arthropathy. J Back Musculoskelet Rehabil 25(2):117–122

26. Wu ZH, Huang NE (2004) A study of the characteristics of white noise using the empirical mode decomposition method. Proce R Soc Lond Ser A: Math, Phys Eng Sci 460(2046): 1597–1611

27. Wu ZH, Huang NE (2009) Ensemble empirical mode decomposition: a noise-assisted data analysis method. Adv Adapt Data Anal 1(1):1–41

28. Wu Y, Krishnan S (2011) Combining least-squares support vector machines for classification of biomedical signals: a case study with knee-joint vibroarthrographic signals. J Exp Theor Artif Intell 23(1):63–77

29. Wu Y, Rangayyan RM (2009) An unbiased linear adaptive filter with normalized coefficients for the removal of noise in electrocardiographic signals. Int J Cogn Inform Nat Intell 3(4): 73–90

30. Wu Y, Rangayyan RM (2011) Noise Cancellation in ECG Signals with an Unbiased Adaptive Filter. In: Wang YX (ed) Transdisciplinary advancements in cognitive mechanisms and human information processing. IGI Global, Hershey, pp 348–366

31. Wu Y, Rangayyan RM, Zhou Y, Ng SC (2009) Filtering electrocardiographic signals using an unbiased and normalized adaptive noise reduction system. Med Eng Phy 31(1):17–26

32. Wu Y, Krishnan S, Rangayyan RM (2010) Computer-aided diagnosis of knee-joint disorders via vibroarthrographic signal analysis: a review. Crit Rev Biomed Eng 38(2):201–224

33. Wu Y, Cai S, Xu F, Shi L, Krishnan S (2012) Chondromalacia patellae detection by analysis of intrinsic mode functions in knee joint vibration signals. In: IFMBE proceedings of 2012 world congress on medical physics and biomedical engineering, Beijing, vol 39, pp 493–496

34. Wu Y, Cai S, Yang S, Zheng F, Xiang N (2013b) Classification of knee joint vibration signals using bivariate feature distribution estimation and maximal posterior probability decision criterion. Entropy 15(4):1375–1387

35. Wu Y, Yang S, Zheng F, Cai S, Lu M, Wu M (2014) Removal of artifacts in knee joint vibroarthrographic signals using ensemble empirical mode decomposition and detrended fluctuation analysis. Physiol Meas 35(3):429–439

36. Zhang YT, Frank CB, Rangayyan RM, Bell GD, Ladly KO (1991) Step size optimization of nonstationary adaptive filtering for knee sound analysis. Med Biol Eng Comput 29(Suppl 2):836

37. Zhang YT, Frank CB, Rangayyan RM, Bell GD (1992) A comparative study of vibromyography and electromyography obtained simultaneously from active human quadriceps. IEEE Trans Biomed Eng 39(10):1045–1052

38. Zhang YT, Frank CB, Rangayyan RM, Bell GD (1992) Mathematical modeling and spectrum analysis of the physiological patello-femoral pulse train produced by slow knee movement. IEEE Trans Biomed Eng 39(9):971–979

39. Zhang YT, Rangayyan RM, Frank CB, Bell GD (1994) Adaptive cancellation of muscle contraction interference from knee joint vibration signals. IEEE Trans Biomed Eng 41(2):181–191

Chapter 3
Signal Analysis

Abstract This chapter provides an overview of the knee joint vibroarthrographic signal analysis methods, including the spatiotemporal analysis, time-frequency analysis, and statistical analysis. The spatiotemporal analysis concentrates on the morphological description of waveform complexity and the detection of physiological or pathological events in the time scale. The time-frequency analysis investigates the time-varying spectral contents in the signal. The statistical analysis focuses on the statistical characteristics and nonlinear dynamics of the nonstationary VAG signal.

3.1 Spatiotemporal Analysis

The commonly used spatiotemporal analysis methods include fixed-window or adaptive segmentation, filtering techniques, signal variability measures, and so forth. The purpose of segmentation is to split the inherently nonstationary VAG signals into several stationary or quasi-stationary segments over a limited time span, so that conventional temporal techniques can be applied to the analysis of the VAG signal segments. Signal segmentation can be performed with a fixed window or adaptive style. In the field of signal processing, fixed segmentation is frequently used for speech processing [20], and adaptive segmentation is well-suited for the analysis of nonstationary biomedical signals such as the electroencephalogram (EEG) [1, 21]. In the case of VAG signal analysis, adaptive segmentation is a better choice than fixed segmentation, because the segmentation with constant-length windows may cause redundancy in the segments of interest, and would also result in poor identification of sudden variations [9, 17, 32].

Tavathia et al. [32] applied a 25th-order linear prediction model to estimate the power spectral density of the VAG signal. The spectral variations of each signal can be computed in terms of the error of the linear prediction model. A reference window of 128 samples is used to determine the length of a signal segment. If the model error is lower than a specific threshold, the current window should be merged with the preceding segment. Such a segment-merging procedure continues until the model error reached the specified threshold level. Then the boundary of the current segment is determined, and a new segment-determination procedure starts with the next 128-sample reference window. The major issue of such a method lies in the

© The Author(s) 2015
Y. Wu, *Knee Joint Vibroarthrographic Signal Processing and Analysis*,
SpringerBriefs in Bioengineering, DOI 10.1007/978-3-662-44284-5_3

definition of the reference window of an appropriate length to suit a specific VAG signal. For example, if a sudden variation occurs in the middle of a window being tested, the segment boundary would be located at the beginning of the window, rather than the exact position of the sudden variation [17].

To overcome the drawback described above, Moussavi et al. [17] proposed an adaptive segmentation method which does not require any reference window. A 5th-order recursive least-squares (RLS) transversal filter with the forgetting factor of 0.98 is used in the segmentation procedure. The signal statistics is measured by computing the squared Euclidean distance between two adjacent tap-weight vectors at each time instant. If the squared Euclidean distance value is over the threshold defined as three times the standard deviation (3 SDs) of the squared Euclidean distance vector, the current time instant is stored in a vector called the primary segment boundaries. The length of 120 samples is chosen as the minimum segment length, which corresponds to approximately 4° of knee flexion or extension motion. The minimum segment length is used to compare the adjacent elements of the primary segment boundary vector; segments of time span smaller than the limit are merged with the adjacent segments.

Krishnan et al. [9] modified the adaptive segmentation procedure of Moussavi et al. [17] as follows. The RLS transversal filter is replaced by an RLS lattice filter. The filter parameter in terms of a conversion factor is utilized to measure the stationarity of the segment being tested, and the threshold is fixed at 0.9985, which is not a variable any longer. The approach of Krishnan et al. [9] simplifies the primary segment boundary detection procedure with the conversion factor and the fixed threshold. In comparison with the RLS transversal filter proposed by Moussavi et al. [17], the lattice filter is self-orthogonalized and possesses the superior properties of modularity, speed of adaptation, and ease of testing for the minimum phase condition [5], such that it is more feasible for hardware implementation of the adaptive segmentation procedure. Figure 3.1 shows the adjacent VAG segment boundaries determined by the RLS lattice method [25]. The segments marked as "1" are associated with a "click" sound heard during auscultation, and the rest of the segments are considered as silent (no sound) segments.

Adaptive segmentation methods are also useful for feature computing and signal classifications. Based on the signal segments, a set of features can be computed to distinguish between the normal and pathological VAG signals. The signal segments can also be annotated with the corresponding attributes, e.g., historically silent or noisy for normal signals; arthroscopically normal or abnormal for pathological signals [17, 25]. Tavathia et al. [32] considered the coefficients and the first dominant pole of the linear prediction model, together with the spectral power ratio, as discriminant features. The first dominant pole was defined at the pole possessing the highest product of its integrated spectral power and radius in the z-plane. The spectral power ratio was defined as the ratio of the fraction of the segment power in the band 40–120 Hz to the total segment power. Moussavi et al. [17] applied a 40th-order forward-backward linear prediction model to analyze the segments. They used total 40 model coefficients, top 10 dominant poles (determined with the same criterion as that used by Tavathia et al. [32]), variance of the means of

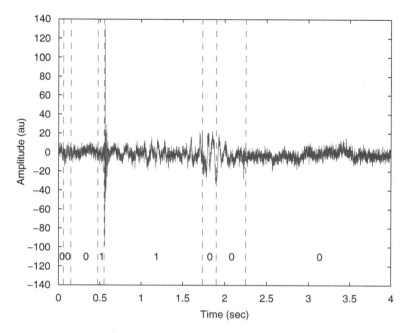

Fig. 3.1 Segments of the vibroarthrographic (VAG) signals recorded from a historically normal subject. The segments annotated as "1" correspond to a "click" sound heard during auscultation, and the rest of the "0" segments are considered as silent (no sound) segments. The *vertical lines* represent segment boundaries determined by the recursive least-squares lattice method. *au*: uncalibrated acceleration units

the segments, and some clinical parameters, to construct the feature set for VAG signal classification. Rangayyan et al. [25] used a 40th-order autoregressive model for parametric representation of the segments. Besides the variance of means of the segments and the clinical parameters used by Moussavi et al. [17], the set of extracted features contained the first six autoregressive coefficients, the first six cepstral coefficients obtained from the power series expansion of the natural logarithm of the autoregressive transfer function, and six dominant poles (with the largest distance values from the origin in the complex z-plane).

The results of previous studies [9, 17, 25, 32] indicated that the features extracted from particular signal segments may provide discriminant information on VAG patterns, which demonstrates the merits of adaptive segmentation for VAG signal analysis. However, a common drawback of the segmentation-based approaches is that they rely on the clinical information obtained during arthroscopy, to annotate the segments of VAG signals. However, it is difficult to define joint angles accurately during arthroscopy, due to the presence of drapes and surgical equipment [10].

Recently, the related studies [22, 23] on spatiotemporal analysis of VAG signals have diverted to the morphological description of waveform complexity. Rangayyan and Wu [22] computed the temporal variations of the VAG signal, in terms of form factor (FF). FF was first introduced by Hjorth [6] to study the variability or "busyness" of EEG signals. The FF value can be computed with the *activity* and *mobility* parameters [21]. The *activity* parameter is defined as the variance σ_x^2 of the given signal x. The *mobility* parameter, M_x, is computed as the square root of the ratio of the variance of the first derivative x' of the signal over the variance of the original signal, i.e.,

$$M_x = \left[\frac{\sigma_{x'}^2}{\sigma_x^2} \right]^{\frac{1}{2}} = \frac{\sigma_{x'}}{\sigma_x}. \tag{3.1}$$

Then, the mathematical definition of FF is the ratio of the mobility of the first derivative of the signal over the mobility of the original signal, which can be expressed as

$$\text{FF} = \frac{M_{x'}}{M_x} = \frac{\sigma_{x''}/\sigma_{x'}}{\sigma_{x'}/\sigma_x}, \tag{3.2}$$

where σ_x, σ_x', and σ_x'' represent the standard deviation (SD) of the signal x, the first derivative x', and the second derivative x'', respectively. For a pure sinusoid signal, its FF value equals to 1. The FF value increases with the extent of the signal complexity. However, because the definition of FF is computed based upon the variances of the first and second derivatives of a given signal, the value of FF could be sensitive to noise.

In addition to the FF, Rangayyan and Wu [23] proposed the variance of the mean-squared (VMS) values in order to measure the local variations of a given VAG signal. The VMS values are computed in the nonoverlapping fixed-duration segments of 5 ms each for the VAG signal. For the VAG signal sampled at 2 kHz, the fixed-length window involves 10 samples. Figure 3.2 displays the VMS results of the VAG signal of a healthy subject. The amplitude of the VAG signal has been normalized by the extreme (maximum absolute value) of the signal. Figure 3.3b illustrates the VMS values computed for the amplitude-normalized VAG signal given in Fig. 3.3a, which was recorded from a symptomatic patient with chondromalacia patellae. It can be observed that the VMS values, which corresponds to the variance of the signal segment power, are remarkably different between the normal and pathological VAG signals. Except for the largest VMS value in correspondence with the "click" event that occurs at around 0.74 s, most of the VMS values are smaller than 0.01 for the normal VAG signal shown in Fig. 3.2. For the abnormal VAG signal in Fig. 3.3, on the other hand, a number of VMS values in relation to the pathological conditions are larger than 0.05 in normalized amplitude. The VMS parameter can also be used to measure the signal variations for a half (with regard to a single knee flexion or extension motion) of the VAG signal. The study of Rangayyan and Wu [23] reported the significant difference (two-sample Student's t-test: $p < 0.01$) of VMS values between the healthy signal group and pathological signal group. Yang et al. [44] measured the fractal scaling index parameter and the averaged envelope amplitude to describe the subtle fluctuations in

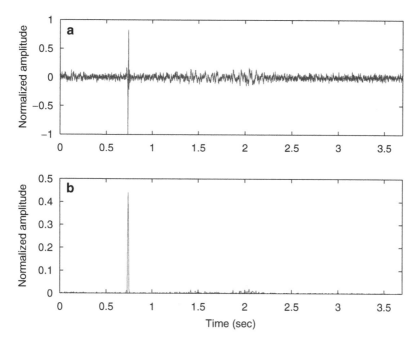

Fig. 3.2 (**a**) The amplitude-normalized vibroarthrographic (VAG) signal of a healthy subject. (**b**) Variations of the mean-squared (VMS) values of the signal computed with the nonoverlapping segments of the fixed 5 ms duration (window length of 10 samples, when signal sampled at 2 kHz)

VAG signals. The Kolmogorov-Smirnov test results indicate that both of the fractal scaling index ($p = 0.0001$) and averaged envelope amplitude ($p = 0.0001$) features are significantly different between the normal and pathological signal groups.

The signal variability over a certain threshold can be measured with the turns count (TC) parameter, which accumulates the number of significant changes in direction for a given signal. A signal turn is commonly identified in a give time series if the data sample simultaneously satisfies the following two conditions [23, 38, 39, 42]:

- It represents an alteration in direction in the signal, i.e., a change in the sign of the derivative;
- The difference (absolute value) between the amplitude of the current alteration and that of the preceding alteration is greater than a threshold.

The total number of the signal turns computed over the time series indicates the degree of fluctuation dynamics in the signal. Such a parameter was first proposed by Willison [36] for analysis of EMG signals related to myopathy. The experiments of Willison suggested that the EMG signal of a patient with myopathy possesses more signal turns than that recorded from a healthy subject at a comparable level of muscular activity [36].

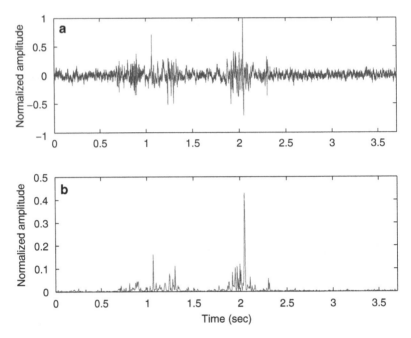

Fig. 3.3 (a) The amplitude-normalized vibroarthrographic (VAG) signal of a patient with chondromalacia patellae. (b) Variations of the mean-squared (VMS) values of the signal computed with the nonoverlapping segments of the fixed 5 ms duration (window length of 10 samples, when signal sampled at 2 kHz)

The identification of significant turns in a given signal, $\{x(i)\}, i = 1, 2, \cdots, I$, contains two steps:

1. **Signal turn detection**: data sample $x(i)$ is included in the turn sequence $\{s(k)\}$, if $[x(i) - x(i-1)][x(i+1) - x(i)] < 0,\ 2 \le i \le I - 1$;
2. **Significant turn identification**: the turn $s(k)$ is selected if the difference between itself and the previous turn is over an assigned threshold level Th, i.e., $|s(k) - s(k-1)| \ge Th$; otherwise $s(k)$ should be removed from the turn sequence.

The threshold level can be predefined with the fixed or adaptive style [2, 23]. Figure 3.4 plots the significant turns identified with the fixed threshold of 0.2 in the segments of the amplitude-normalized VAG signals. It is clear that the number of signal turns detected in the pathological VAG signal segment is larger than that of the normal VAG signal segment. The degree of complexity in the pathological VAG signal has increased because the degenerative articular surface due to chondromalacia patellae results in more friction and contacts between the cartilages.

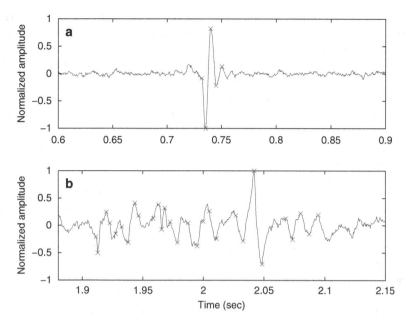

Fig. 3.4 (**a**) The signal turns identified in the time span range from 0.6 to 0.9 s of the amplitude-normalized vibroarthrographic signal of a healthy subject. (**b**) The signal turns identified in the time span range from 1.9 to 2.1 s of the amplitude-normalized vibroarthrographic signal of a patient with chondromalacia patellae. The significant signal turns over the fixed threshold of 0.2 are marked with *crosses*

3.2 Time-Frequency Analysis

The information about the inherent rhythms and periodicity of a given VAG signal can be readily expressed and analyzed in the frequency domain. The frequency analysis of biomedical signals are often performed with the Fourier transform that is able to transform signals between time domain and frequency domain [21]. For VAG signal analysis, Ladly et al. [12] demonstrated clear separation between VAG signals of normal knees and injured knees with articular cartilage damage using the signal power and median frequency measures. After averaging the VAG signals over the total knee flexion-to-extension cycles, Ladly et al. [12] reported up to 112 % difference in mean signal power and up to 173 % difference in median frequency between normal and pathological VAG signals. In the last 60° of knee extension, the differences increased to 471 % in mean power and 652 % in median frequency between normal and pathological signals. The study of Ladly et al. [12] indicated the evidence that VAG signals can be separated in terms of their power and median frequency in the angle range from 60–0°. Tanaka and Hoshiyama [31] applied the fast Fourier transform with a Hamming window of 4,096 samples to the 145 VAG signals recorded from 99 healthy control knees and 46 knees with osteoarthritis during standing-up and sitting-down movements. Their study [31] suggested that the mean frequency of power spectrum at 50–99 and 100–149 Hz of the VAG signals in knee osteoarthritis is significantly greater (Tukey-Kramer test: $p < 0.001$) than that of the healthy control signals.

The major disadvantage of the frequency analysis is that such a method cannot accurately describe the varying frequency components in response to the elapsed time [2]. For the VAG signal that is inherent nonstationary and with time-varying spectral properties, time-frequency distribution (TFD) analysis methods can overcome the drawbacks of the frequency-based approaches [3]. The matching pursuit (MP) algorithm proposed by Mallat and Zhang [14] is a prevailing technique to decompose the signal using basis functions with good time-frequency properties (referred to as atoms).

The MP method is a so-called "greedy" algorithm that successively approximates a signal $x(t)$ of N samples with orthogonal projections onto elements from a waveform dictionary $\mathscr{D} = \{d_r(t)\}_{r\in\Gamma}$ of P vectors, in which $\|d_r\| = \sqrt{\left[\int d_r^2(t)dt\right]} = 1$. Gabor function, local cosine trees, and wavelet packets are often applied to build up dictionaries for MP applications. The Daubechies wavelets are excellent choice for the VAG signal decomposition using the MP algorithm [2], because they belong to a family of orthogonal wavelets that have a support of minimum size for any given number of vanishing moments [4]. Based on the Daubechies wavelets, the MP algorithm may decompose a given signal with appropriate time and scale properties [13].

The projection of VAG signal $x(t)$ using the dictionary of wavelet packet bases, $d_{r_m}(t)$, calculated with a Daubechies wavelet filter, can be formulated as

$$x(t) = \sum_{m=0}^{M-1} a_m d_{r_m}(t), \tag{3.3}$$

where a_m are the expansion coefficients and M denotes the iterations of decomposition. And the wavelet MP decomposition can be implemented as follows: In the beginning, $x(t)$ is projected on a vector $d_{r_0}(t) \in \mathscr{D}$ and the residue $R^1 x(t)$ is computed, i.e.,

$$x(t) = \langle x, d_{r_0}\rangle d_{r_0}(t) + R^1 x(t), \tag{3.4}$$

where $\langle x, d_{r_0}\rangle$ denotes the inner product (projection). Since the first atom $d_{r_0}(t)$ is orthogonal to $R^1 x(t)$, we have

$$\|x\|^2 = |\langle x, d_{r_0}\rangle|^2 + \|R^1 x\|^2. \tag{3.5}$$

In order to minimize $\|R^1 x\|$, $r_0 \in \Gamma$ is chosen such that $|\langle x, d_{r_0}\rangle|$ is maximum, i.e.,

$$|\langle x, d_{r_0}\rangle| \geq \sup_{r\in\Gamma} |\langle x, d_r\rangle|. \tag{3.6}$$

The MP iterates this procedure by subdecomposing the residue. And the VAG signal $x(t)$ after M iterations of decomposition is then expressed as

$$x(t) = \sum_{m=1}^{M-1} \langle R^m x, \ d_{r_m} \rangle \, d_{r_m}(t) + R^M x(t), \tag{3.7}$$

where $|\langle x, \ d_{r_m} \rangle| \geq \sup\limits_{r \in \Gamma} |\langle x, \ d_r \rangle|$ and $R^0 x(t) \equiv x(t)$. There are three ways to stop the iterative MP decomposition process. A straightforward way is to predefine the number M of the time-frequency atoms. Such a practice is somewhat arbitrary because the results much depend on personal experience. The second approach to end the iterative process is according to the convergence of residual energy, $\|R^m x\|^2$, because the residue term $R^M x(t)$ can be regarded as noise after sufficient iterations [8, 10]. Cai et al. [2] suggested using the signal-to-noise ratio (SNR) indicator to determine the MP decomposition, i.e., the decomposition process is terminated if the SNR reaches a particular level. With a given SNR threshold, the number of the wavelet MP decomposition iterations for a pathological VAG signal would be larger than that for a normal signal, because the pathological signal is much more complex and also contaminated by a larger amount of artifacts such as muscle contraction interference [2].

Figure 3.5 displays a pair samples of knee joint VAG signals recorded from a healthy subject and a symptomatic patient with chondromalacia patellae. Based on

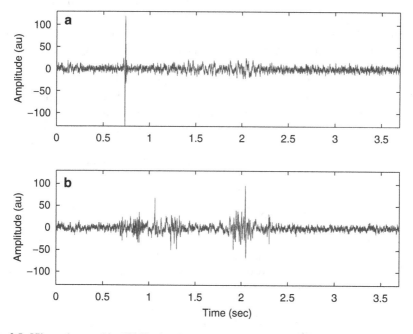

Fig. 3.5 Vibroarthrographic (VAG) signal examples recorded from (**a**) a healthy adult (male, 40 years old); (**b**) of a symptomatic patient (male, 33 years old) with Grade II and III chondromalacia patellae. *au*: uncalibrated acceleration units

the decomposition ending criterion in reference to the SNR threshold of 15 dB [2], the MP algorithm with the Daubechies 8 wavelet dictionary would produce 774 atoms for the normal signal in Fig. 3.5a, and 534 atoms for the pathological signal in Fig. 3.5b, respectively. Their corresponding MP TFD illustrations are plotted in Fig. 3.6, where the density of each MP atom is proportional to the coefficient value. It can be observed that the normal and pathological VAG signals have very different spatial patterns in the time-frequency plane. For the normal VAG signal in Fig. 3.6a, most of the MP atoms with large coefficient value fall within the frequency band of 0–400 Hz. On the other hand, the dominant MP atoms of the pathological signal mainly congregate in the time spans from 0.6 to 1.4 s and from 1.8 to 2.1 s, and occupy a broader frequency band from 0 to 1,000 Hz.

The short-time Fourier transform (STFT) is also very useful for characterization of the frequency distribution of signal segments in the transient time spans [18]. Figure 3.7 provides the STFT spectrograms of the VAG signals in Fig. 3.5. The spectrograms were computed using the fast Fourier transform (FFT) and the Hamming window in the length of 128 samples, with the overlapping segment length of 120 samples. From Fig. 3.8, it can be observed that the time-frequency resolution of the STFT TFD illustrations is not good enough to facilitate enhanced feature identification in the VAG signals. On the other hand, the MP TFDs offer a better joint resolution of time-frequency structures both in time and frequency scales, as shown in Fig. 3.6. The atoms provided by the MP algorithm are well-suited for tracking the time-varying power spectral content of the VAG signals [41].

The MP atoms are useful for feature extraction and further pattern classification. Krishnan et al. [10] used the Wigner-Ville distribution of the MP atoms to represent the signal TFD, and the minimum cross-entropy optimization method to modify the TFD to satisfy both the positive and marginal requirements (see Fig. 3.8a for a block diagram of the procedure). The cross-entropy minimization is a general method to infer an unknown probability density function (PDF) when there exists *a priori* estimate of the PDF with a few variable constraints [29]. With the optimized TFD, denoted as $M(t, \omega)$, the time-varying parameters, such as the energy parameter, the energy spread parameter, the frequency parameter, and the frequency spread parameter, can be computed as features for signal classifications [7, 10]. The energy parameter (EP) is the mean of the TFD $M(t, \omega)$ over the frequency range in a time span [10]:

$$\text{EP}(t) = \frac{\sum_{\omega=0}^{\omega_n} M(t, \omega)}{\omega_n}, \tag{3.8}$$

where ω_n is the maximum frequency of the signal. The energy spread parameter (ESP) that describes the spread of energy over frequency for a time span can be computed as the SD of the TFD as [10]

$$\text{ESP}(t) = \left[\frac{\sum_{\omega=0}^{\omega_n} [M(t, \omega) - \text{EP}(t)]^2}{\omega_n} \right]^{\frac{1}{2}}. \tag{3.9}$$

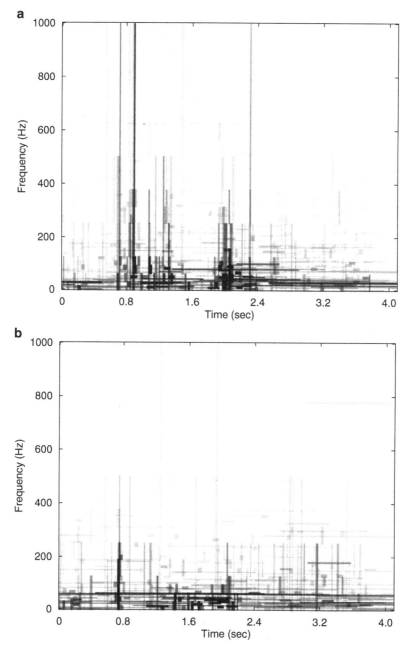

Fig. 3.6 Wavelet matching pursuit atoms of the knee joint vibroarthrographic signals in Fig. 3.5: (**a**) of a healthy subject; (**b**) of a patient with chondromalacia patellae. The dictionary of wavelet packet bases was calculated by a Daubechies 8 filter

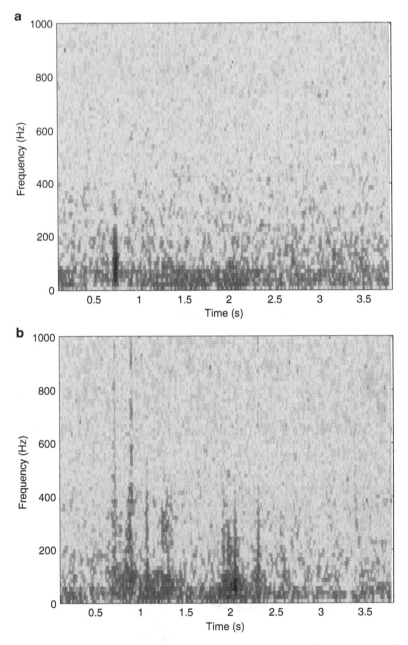

Fig. 3.7 Spectrograms of the knee joint vibroarthrographic signals in Fig. 3.5 computed using the short-time Fourier transform: (**a**) of a healthy subject; (**b**) of a patient with chondromalacia patellae

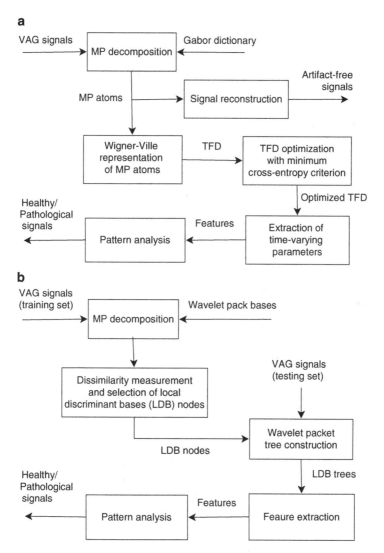

Fig. 3.8 Block diagrams of the knee joint vibroarthrographic (*VAG*) signal analysis based on the matching pursuit (*MP*) algorithm proposed (**a**) by Krishnan et al. [10] and (**b**) by Umapathy et al. [33], respectively. *TFD*: time-frequency distribution; *LDB* local discriminant bases

The frequency parameter (FP) that indicates the instantaneous mean frequency can be computed as the first moment of the TFD in a time span as [10]

$$FP(t) = \frac{\sum_{\omega=0}^{\omega_n} \omega M(t,\omega)}{\sum_{\omega=0}^{\omega_n} M(t,\omega)}. \tag{3.10}$$

The frequency spread parameter (FSP) is the second central moment of the TFD in a time span [10], i.e.,

$$FSP(t) = \left[\frac{\sum_{\omega=0}^{\omega_n} [\omega - FP(t)]^2 M(t, \omega)}{\sum_{\omega=0}^{\omega_n} M(t, \omega)} \right]^{\frac{1}{2}}. \tag{3.11}$$

Based on the wavelet MP decomposition, Umapathy and Krishnan [33] used the local discriminant bases (LDB) algorithms to construct wavelet packet LDB trees at different levels, and then computed three dissimilarity measures to select 15 LDB tree nodes that maximized the inter-class dissimilarity for VAG signal classification (see Fig. 3.8b for the corresponding block diagram).

In general, The MP algorithm is well-suited for analysis of nonstationary VAG signals, because the MP atoms can clearly display the time-frequency characteristics of the signals. The disadvantage of the MP algorithm is concerned with its computational complexity. For a wavelet packet dictionary that contains $P = N \log_2 N$ vectors, a single MP iteration requires $O(N \log_2 N)$ operations [13]. For the VAG data illustrated in Fig. 3.5, each signal consists of $N = f_s \times T = 8,000$ samples, and the MP decomposition becomes computationally expensive [37].

3.3   Statistical Analysis

The statistical parameters can help provide the variant information about the VAG signal [24]. To derive the statistical parameters, the histogram is necessary as a reference of the probability density function (PDF) of a given signal. The histogram is often estimated with B bins, which helped calculate the probability of occurrence with B containers of equal length in the amplitude range of the signal. The number of bins is essential for an accurate estimate of the histogram. Scott [27] suggested that the optimal choice of bin number should help minimize the mean-squared error between the estimated histogram and the Gaussian PDF, which can be obtained as

$$B = \lceil \frac{(y_{max} - y_{min})}{3.49 \, s \, n^{-1/3}} \rceil \tag{3.12}$$

where s and n represent the SD and the number of samples in the VAG signal, respectively; y_{max} and y_{min} are the highest and lowest amplitude values of the signal, respectively; and the operator $\lceil \cdot \rceil$ rounds the number of bins toward the nearest integer greater than or equal to it.

The PDF can be estimated from a collection of signal samples by using the nonparametric Parzen window method [19]. Assume that a signal contains a set of K samples, $\{y_k\}, k = 1, 2, \cdots, K$, with an unknown underlying PDF $p(y)$. The estimated PDF $\hat{p}(y)$ can be expressed as [24, 39, 40, 43]

$$\hat{p}(y) = \frac{1}{K} \sum_{k=1}^{K} w(y - y_k),$$

(3.13)

where $w(\cdot)$ represents a window function that integrates to unity. The Gaussian window can be used as the window function as [24]

$$w(y - y_k) = \frac{1}{\sigma_P \sqrt{2\pi}} \exp\left[-\frac{(y - y_k)^2}{2\sigma_P^2}\right],$$

(3.14)

where σ_P denotes the spread parameter that determines the width of a Gaussian window, with the center located at y_k. The spread parameter of the Parzen-window PDF should be optimized with the same resolution as the histogram, i.e., the estimated probability density, $\hat{p}(y^b)$, $b = 1, 2, \cdots, B$, was also represented with B bins [43]. The optimization of spread parameter can be achieved by minimizing the mean-squared error (MSE) between the Parzen-window PDF, $\hat{p}(y^b)$, and the histogram, $\hat{h}(y^b)$, i.e.,

$$\min\left\{\frac{1}{B} \sum_{b=1}^{B} [\hat{p}(y^b) - \hat{h}(y^b)]^2\right\}.$$

(3.15)

Figure 3.9 provides the histogram, the Gaussian fit, and the Parzen-window PDFs for the healthy subject group (averaged over the 51 healthy adults) and for the pathological group (averaged over the 38 patients with knee joint disorders) [24]. The amplitude of each VAG signal has been normalized to the range from 0 to 1.

The statistical parameters, such as mean (μ), variance (σ^2), skewness (SK), kurtosis (KU), and entropy, can be computed based on the estimated PDF of the VAG signal [22–24]. The calculations of mean and variance parameters are expressed as

$$\mu = \sum_{b=1}^{B} y^b \hat{p}(y^b),$$

(3.16)

and

$$\sigma^2 = \sum_{b=1}^{B} (y^b - \mu)^2 \hat{p}(y^b).$$

(3.17)

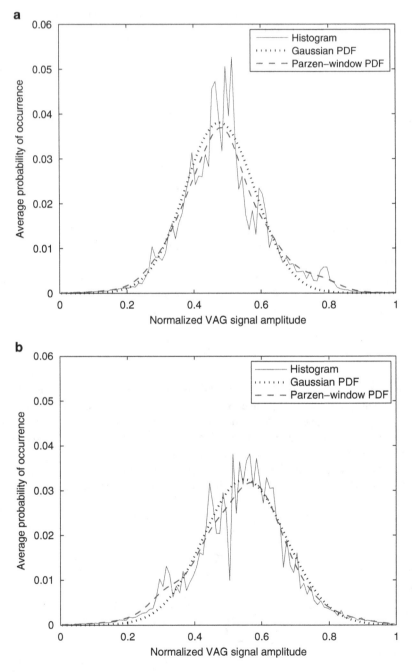

Fig. 3.9 The averaged histogram, the Gaussian fit, and the nonparametric Parzen-window estimates of the probability density functions of VAG signals: (**a**) for healthy adults; (**b**) for patients with knee joint pathology. The amplitude of VAG signals has been normalized to the range from 0 to 1 (Reprinted with permission from Ref. [24]. © 2010 Elsevier)

The SK and KU are two parameters which are usually used to measure the asymmetry and "peakedness" of the PDF. The SK and KU can be calculated as the third and fourth normalized moments of the PDF [16, 21, 24, 43], given by

$$SK = \frac{m_3}{(m_2)^{3/2}},$$ (3.18)

and

$$KU = \frac{m_4}{(m_2)^2},$$ (3.19)

where m_i denotes the ith central moment of the PDF, defined by

$$m_i = \sum_{b=1}^{B} (y^b - \mu)^i \, \hat{p}(y^b).$$ (3.20)

Figure 3.10 displays three typical SK parameters for the unimodal PDFs [43]: if the PDF is symmetric or balanced, e.g., the Gaussian distribution, the skewness

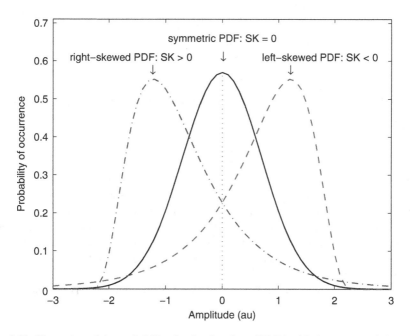

Fig. 3.10 Illustration of the probability density functions (*PDFs*) with three types of skewness (*SK*): right-skewed PDF, *dash-dot curve*, SK > 0; symmetric PDF, *solid curve*, SK = 0 (in particular Gaussian distributions); left-skewed PDF, *dashed curve*, SK < 0. *Dot line* represents a central axis up to the mean of the symmetric PDF. *au*: arbitrary units (Reprinted with permission from Ref. [43])

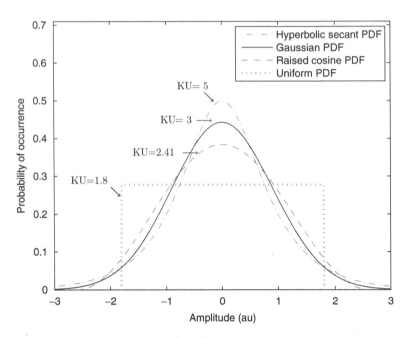

Fig. 3.11 Illustration of four typical probability density functions (*PDFs*), which possess different kurtosis (*KU*) values: uniform distribution, *dot curve*, KU = 1.8; raised cosine distribution, *dashed curve*, KU = 2.41; Gaussian distribution, *solid curve*, KU = 3; hyperbolic secant distribution, *dash-dot curve*, KU = 5. *au*: arbitrary units (Reprinted with permission from Ref. [43])

is zero; if the mass of the PDF is concentrated on the left of the mean, the PDF is right-skewed such that the skewness is positive (SK > 0); in contrast, if the mass of the PDF concentrates on the right of the mean, the PDF is then left-skewed so that the skewness is negative (SK < 0).

Figure 3.11 plots four well-known PDFs with different KU values. It is worth noting that the sharper the peak of distribution, the larger the KU becomes [43]. The top of uniform distribution is flat, and its KU is smallest (KU = 1.8); the Gaussian distribution possesses a KU value of 3.0, which is usually considered as the benchmark for KU comparison; the peak of the raised cosine PDF is more rounded than the Gaussian distribution, so that the KU value equals to 2.41; the hyperbolic secant PDF [30] has the sharpest peak and the largest KU value (KU = 5) among these four distributions.

As defined in Shannon's information theory [28], entropy (H) is a statistical parameter to measure the spread of the PDF [24], written as

$$H = -\sum_{b=1}^{B} p(y^b) \log_2 p(y^b).$$ (3.21)

The entropy reaches its maximum value for a uniform PDF. For the PDFs with narrow ranges of substantial probability values, the entropy values are lower. The Kullback–Leibler divergence (KLD), also known as relative entropy, is nonsymmetric parameter that indicates the difference between two PDFs [11]. Given two PDFs $p_1(y^b)$ and $p_2(y^b)$, the KLD of $p_2(y^b)$ from $p_1(y^b)$ measures the information lost when $p_2(y^b)$ is used to approximate $p_1(y^b)$ as

$$\text{KLD}(p_1||p_2) = \sum_{b=1}^{B} p_1(y^b) \ln\left[\frac{p_1(y^b)}{p_2(y^b)}\right]. \tag{3.22}$$

Rangayyan and Wu [24] compared the difference of the KLD between the normal from pathological signal groups based on the estimated Parzen-window PDFs of VAG signals.

The nonlinear dynamics present in the VAG signal can be investigated using the fractal analysis methods [26]. The fractals of a signal describes the self-similarity properties at different scales. For example, the Brownian motion can be described as a typical fractal model with a random walk process $V(t)$ over the time span t. Mandelbrot [15] proposed the fractional Brownian motion (fBm) model, which has been used to generate advanced mathematical models for descriptions of natural fractal scenery. Models based on fBm have been extended to two dimensions for the synthesis of Brownian surfaces and three dimensions to generate Brownian clouds [34]. Figure 3.12 shows four signal examples, $V_{\text{HE}}(t)$, generated based on the fBm model. The scaling of the traces is characterized by the Hurst exponent scaling parameter, HE $(0 \leq \text{HE} \leq 1)$. A relatively smooth signal possess a high value of HE close to 1. In contrast, a small HE value commonly indicates a rougher trace. The variable HE represents the changes in amplitude, $\Delta V = V(t_2) - V(t_1)$, in relation to different temporal duration, $\Delta t = t_2 - t_1$, by the scaling law $\Delta V \propto (\Delta t)^{\text{HE}}$ [35].

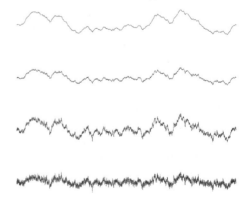

Fig. 3.12 Signal examples generated based on the fractional Brownian motion model for different values of Hurst exponent (HE) and fractal dimension (FD). From top to bottom: model HE = 0.9, 0.6, 0.4, 0.1; model FD = 1.1, 1.4, 1.6, 1.9; estimated FD = 1.104, 1.404, 1.604, 1.903 (Reprinted with permission from Ref. [26]. © 2013 Elsevier)

The zeros-set of a signal is the set of disconnected data points with a topological dimension of zero, D_0, written as [26, 35]

$$D_0 = 1 - HE. \tag{3.23}$$

The fractal dimension (FD) of the signal is then expressed as [26]

$$FD = D_0 + 1 = 2 - HE. \tag{3.24}$$

The power spectral density (PSD), $P_v(f)$, can be used to estimate the power of fluctuations at a specific frequency [26]. The inverse power law or the $1/f$ model is defined as the quantity $V(t)$ with the best linear fitting to its PSD, varying as $1/f^\beta$, in the double logarithmic plane [26]. The PSD of a self-affine fBm signal in an E-dimensional Euclidean space satisfies the power law, $P_v(f) \propto 1/f^\beta$, with the FD value computed as

$$FD = E + 1 - HE, \tag{3.25}$$

where

$$HE = \frac{\beta - 1}{2}. \tag{3.26}$$

The FD with respect to the spectral component β for the VAG signal ($E = 1$) is given by

$$FD = \frac{5 - \beta}{2}. \tag{3.27}$$

For the VAG signal analysis, Rangayyan et al. [26] applied the discrete Fourier transform with Hanning window PSD estimates to the VAG signal. It is important to choose an appropriate frequency range for the best linear fitting of the PSD. The low-frequency content of the signal corresponds to the slow baseline drift, and the high-frequency components of the VAG signal are often contaminated by muscle contraction artifacts. In the work of Rangayyan et al. [26], the frequency range from 10 to 300 Hz were selected to perform the linear fitting for the VAG signals. Figure 3.13 displays the double logarithmic plots the PSDs estimated for the VAG signals recorded from a healthy subject and a patient with knee joint pathology. The FD values computed according to the linear fitting lines of the PSDs are 1.801 and 1.319 for the normal and pathological signals, respectively. The statistics of the FD parameters are 1.8061±0.2398 and 1.6695±0.2226 for the healthy and pathological signal groups, respectively. To study the nonlinear dynamics of the VAG signal, Rangayyan et al. [26] also computed the FD values for every single quarter segment of the VAG signal, and then used these FD features for signal classifications.

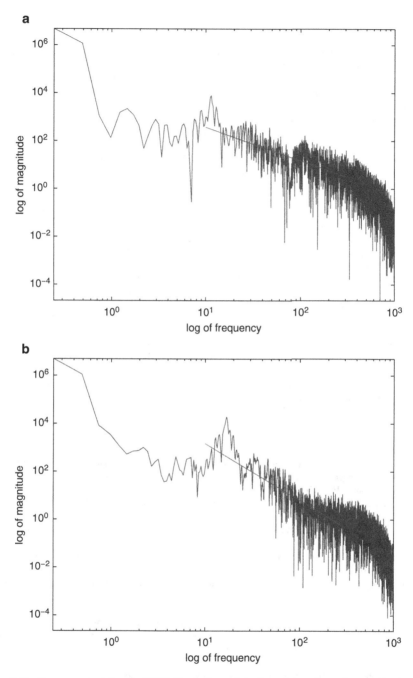

Fig. 3.13 Power spectral density (PSD) illustrations of the knee joint vibroarthrographic signals with the linear fitting in the range from 10 to 300 Hz: (**a**) of a healthy subject (fractal dimension: 1.801); (**b**) of a patient with knee joint pathology (fractal dimension: 1.319) (Reprinted with permission from Ref. [26]. © 2013 Elsevier)

References

1. Barlow JS, Creutzfeldt OD, Michael D, Houchin J, Epelbaum H (1981) Automatic adaptive segmentation of clinical EEGs. Electroencephalogr Clin Neurophysiol 51(5):512–525
2. Cai S, Yang S, Zheng F, Lu M, Wu Y, Krishnan S (2013) Knee joint vibration signal analysis with matching pursuit decomposition and dynamic weighted classifier fusion. Comput Math Methods Med 2013:Article ID 904267
3. Cohen L (1989) Time-frequency distributions: a review. Proc IEEE 77(7):941–981
4. Daubechies I (1990) The wavelet transform time-frequency localization and signal analysis. IEEE Trans Inf Theory 36(5):961–1005
5. Haykin S (2002) Adaptive filter theory, 4th edn. Prentice Hall PTR, Englewood Cliffs
6. Hjorth B (1973) The physical significance of time domain descriptors in EEG analysis. Electroencephalogr Clin Neurophysiol 34(3):321–325
7. Kim KS, Seo JH, Kang JU, Song CG (2009) An enhanced algorithm for knee joint sound classification using feature extraction based on time-frequency analysis. Comput Methods Progr Biomed 94(2):198–206
8. Krishnan S, Rangayyan RM (2000) Automatic de-noising of knee-joint vibration signals using adaptive time-frequency representations. Med Biol Eng Comput 38(8):2–8
9. Krishnan S, Rangayyan RM, Bell GD, Frank CB, Ladly KO (1997) Adaptive filtering, modelling, and classification of knee joint vibroarthrographic signals for non-invasive diagnosis of articular cartilage pathology. Med Biol Eng Comput 35(6):677–684
10. Krishnan S, Rangayyan RM, Bell GD, Frank CB (2000) Adaptive time-frequency analysis of knee joint vibroarthrographic signals for noninvasive screening of articular cartilage pathology. IEEE Trans Biomed Eng 47(6):773–783
11. Kullback S, Leibler RA (1951) On information and sufficiency. Ann Math Stat 22(1):79–86
12. Ladly KO, Frank CB, Bell GD, Zhang YT, Rangayyan RM (1993) The effect of external loads and cyclic loading on normal patellofemoral joint signals. Def Sci J 43:201–210
13. Mallat S (1999) A wavelet tour of signal processing, 2nd edn. Academic, San Diego
14. Mallat S, Zhang Z (1993) Matching pursuits with time-frequency dictionaries. IEEE Trans Signal Process 41(12):3397–3415
15. Mandelbrot BB (1983) The fractal geometry of nature. W. H. Freeman, San Francisco
16. Marques de Sa JP (2003) Applied statistics using SPSS, STATISTICA, and MATLAB. Springer, Berlin
17. Moussavi ZMK, Rangayyan RM, Bell GD, Frank CB, Ladly KO, Zhang YT (1996) Screening of vibroarthrographic signals via adaptive segmentation and linear prediction modeling. IEEE Trans Biomed Eng 43(1):15–23
18. Oppenheim AV, Schafer RW (1989) Discrete-time signal processing. Prentice-Hall, Englewood Cliffs
19. Parzen E (1962) On estimation of a probability density function and mode. Ann Math Stat 33(3):1065–1076
20. Rabiner LR, Schafer RW (1978) Digital processing of speech signals. Prentice-Hall PTR, Englewood Cliffs
21. Rangayyan RM (2002) Biomedical signal analysis: a case-study approach. IEEE/Wiley, New York
22. Rangayyan RM, Wu YF (2008) Screening of knee-joint vibroarthrographic signals using statistical parameters and radial basis functions. Med Biol Eng Comput 46(3):223–232
23. Rangayyan RM, Wu Y (2009) Analysis of vibroarthrographic signals with features related to signal variability and radial-basis functions. Ann Bio Eng 37(1):156–163
24. Rangayyan RM, Wu Y (2010) Screening of knee-joint vibroarthrographic signals using probability density functions estimated with Parzen windows. Biomed Signal Process Control 5(1): 53–58

25. Rangayyan RM, Krishnan S, Bell GD, Frank CB, Ladly KO (1997) Parametric representation and screening of knee joint vibroarthrographic signals. IEEE Trans Biomed Eng 44(11): 1068–1074
26. Rangayyan RM, Oloumi F, Wu Y, Cai S (2013) Fractal analysis of knee-joint vibroarthrographic signals via power spectral analysis. Biomed Signal Process Control 8(1):26–29
27. Scott DW (1979) On optimal and data-based histograms. Biometrika 66(3):605–610
28. Shannon CE (1948) A mathematical theory of communication. Bell Syst Tech J 27:379–423, 623–656
29. Shore J, Johnson R (1981) Properties of cross-entropy minimization. IEEE Trans Inf Theory 27(4):472–482
30. Smyth GK (1994) A note on modelling cross correlations: hyperbolic secant regression. Biometrika 81(2):396–402
31. Tanaka N, Hoshiyama M (2012) Vibroarthrography in patients with knee arthropathy. J Back Musculoskelet Rehabil 25(2):117–122
32. Tavathia S, Rangayyan RM, Frank CB, Bell GD, Ladly KO, Zhang YT (1992) Analysis of knee vibration signals using linear prediction. IEEE Trans Biomed Eng 39(9):959–970
33. Umapathy K, Krishnan S (2006) Modified local discriminant bases algorithm and its application in analysis of human knee joint vibration signals. IEEE Trans Biomed Eng 53(3):517–523
34. Voss RF (1985) Random fractal forgeries. In: Earnshaw RA (ed) Fundamental algorithms for computer graphics. Springer, New York, pp 805–835
35. Voss RF (1988) Fractals in nature: from characterization to simulation. In: Peitgen HO, Saupe D (eds) The science of fractal images. Springer, New York, pp 21–70
36. Willison RG (1964) Analysis of electrical activity in healthy and dystrophic muscle in man. J Neurol Neurosurg Psychiatry 27(5):386–394
37. Wu Y, Krishnan S (2009) Classification of knee-joint vibroarthrographic signals using time-domain and time-frequency domain features and least-squares support vector machine. In: Proceedings of the 16th international conference on digital signal processing, Santorini, pp 361–366
38. Wu Y, Krishnan S (2009) Computer-aided analysis of gait rhythm fluctuations in amyotrophic lateral sclerosis. Med Biol Eng Comput 47(11):1165–1171
39. Wu Y, Krishnan S (2010) Statistical analysis of gait rhythm in patients with Parkinson's disease. IEEE Trans Neural Syst Rehabil Eng 18(2):150–158
40. Wu Y, Shi L (2011) Analysis of altered gait rhythm in amyotrophic lateral sclerosis based on nonparametric probability density function estimation. Med Eng Phys 33(3):347–355
41. Wu Y, Krishnan S, Rangayyan RM (2010) Computer-aided diagnosis of knee-joint disorders via vibroarthrographic signal analysis: a review. Crit Rev Biomed Eng 38(2):201–224
42. Wu Y, Cai S, Xu F, Shi L, Krishnan S (2012) Chondromalacia patellae detection by analysis of intrinsic mode functions in knee joint vibration signals. In: IFMBE proceedings of 2012 world congress on medical physics and biomedical engineering, Beijing, vol 39, pp 493–496
43. Xiang N, Cai S, Yang S, Zhong Z, Zheng F, He J, Wu Y (2013) Statistical analysis of gait maturation in children using nonparametric probability density function modeling. Entropy 15(3):753–766
44. Yang S, Cai S, Zheng F, Wu Y, Liu K, Wu M, Zou Q, Chen J (2014) Representation of fluctuation features in pathological knee joint vibroarthrographic signals using kernel density modeling method. Med Eng Phys 36(10):1305–1311

Chapter 4
Feature Computing and Signal Classifications

Abstract In this chapter, we describe the feature computing and pattern analysis methods for VAG signal classifications. The purpose of feature selection is to study the feature correlations and then exclude the redundant features before pattern classifications. The reduction of feature dimensions may avoid excessive computation expenses, such that the pattern analysis methods based on the most informative features can also achieve favorable classification results. The signal classification methods include Fisher's linear discriminant analysis, radial basis function network, Vapnik and least-squares support vector machines, Bayesian decision rule, and multiple classifier fusion systems. The text also presents the common diagnostic performance techniques such as cross-validation, confusion matrix, and receiver operating characteristic curves. Finally, we review the state-of-the-art methods for the VAG signal classifications and compare the results reported in recent literature.

4.1 Feature Selection and Dimensionality Reduction

In statistical pattern recognition, the data set usually contains some redundant or irrelevant features. The irrelevant features cannot provide useful information for a particular classification task, and those redundant features do not contribute more to the current feature set. It is therefore necessary to perform feature analysis in order to remove the redundant information and reduce the feature dimensions. Given a data set with L features, an exhaustive search of subsets involves $C(L, I)$ combinations for I features. The optimal value of I can be determined by searching for all possible 2^L feature combinations, which is computational expensive and impractical. Instead of global optimality of feature subsets, the sequential search methods that use greedy strategies are able to provide a combination result of selected features with local optimality [10]. The sequential forward selection (SFS) and the sequential backward selection (SBS) are two popular feature selection techniques in the literature. The SFS method proposed by Whitney [39] starts with an empty feature set and sequentially adds one feature at a time. Once a feature is retained in the SFS selected subset, it cannot be discarded in the next searching step. The SBS method introduced by Marill and Green [21] is the opposite-direction searching algorithm, which begins with all available features and sequentially

© The Author(s) 2015
Y. Wu, *Knee Joint Vibroarthrographic Signal Processing and Analysis*,
SpringerBriefs in Bioengineering, DOI 10.1007/978-3-662-44284-5_4

excludes one feature that makes least contribution to the criterion function at a time. In general, the SBS method would occupy more computation resources than the SFS approach. The evaluation criterion is important for the effectiveness of feature selection. In machine learning, the selected features are usually evaluated by the cross-validation method. In statistics, the logistic regression [5] can be employed in the feature selection process to evaluate the performance, although such a criterion may sometimes cause the inherent problem of nesting.

4.2   Fisher's Linear Discriminant Analysis

Fisher's linear discriminant analysis (FLDA) is a simple but effective pattern classi-fication tool that searches a mapping orientation which leads to the best separation among the classes [8]. The FLDA works by projecting the multidimensional data onto a linear surface such that the dimensionality of the complex data set can be reduced [15]. The major advantage of the FLDA is that it does not require the prior assumption about the distribution of input patterns. It is slightly different from the linear discriminant analysis that assumes that the classes are with normal distributions or equal covariances [23].

The linear discriminant function produces the linear decision surface to separate the patterns with L-dimensional features as

$$y = \sum_{l=1}^{L} w_l f_l + w_0, \qquad (4.1)$$

where w_l is the appropriate weights that indicates linear projection direction and w_0 is the bias. We may define the $(L+1)$-by-1 input feature vector $\mathbf{f} = [+1, f_1, f_2, \cdots, f_L]^T$ and the $(L+1)$-by-1 weight vector $\mathbf{w} = [w_0, w_1, w_2, \cdots, w_L]^T$, such that the linear discriminant function can also be written as

$$y = \mathbf{w}^T \mathbf{f}. \qquad (4.2)$$

The objective of the FLDA algorithm is to seek a linear combination of features that yields the maximization of the discriminant function [5, 45]:

$$J(\mathbf{w}) = \frac{\mathbf{w}^T \mathbf{S}_B \mathbf{w}}{\mathbf{w}^T \mathbf{S}_W \mathbf{w}}, \qquad (4.3)$$

where $\mathbf{S}_B$ represents the inter-class (or between-class) scatter matrix, and $\mathbf{S}_W$ denotes the intra-class (or within-class) scatter matrix. For the binary classification of the knee joint VAG signals, the scatter matrices $\mathbf{S}_B$ and $\mathbf{S}_W$ are defined as [23, 45]:

$$\mathbf{S}_B = (\mathbf{m}_N - \mathbf{m}_A)(\mathbf{m}_N - \mathbf{m}_A)^T, \qquad (4.4)$$

and

$$\mathbf{S}_W = \sum_{\mathbf{u} \in \omega_N} (\mathbf{u} - \mathbf{m_N})(\mathbf{u} - \mathbf{m_N})^T + \sum_{\mathbf{u} \in \omega_A} (\mathbf{u} - \mathbf{m_A})(\mathbf{u} - \mathbf{m_A})^T, \qquad (4.5)$$

where $\mathbf{m_N}$ and $\mathbf{m_A}$ denote the mean values of $\mathbf{u}$ for the normal and abnormal signal groups, respectively. The discriminant function $J(\mathbf{w})$ can be maximized by the Lagrange multiplier method, if the intra-class scatter matrix $\mathbf{S}_W$ is nonsingular [5]. The projection direction that makes the best linear separation of the input patterns is given by the solution $\mathbf{w}^* = \mathbf{S}_W^{-1}(\mathbf{m_N} - \mathbf{m_A})$ [45].

4.3 Radial Basis Function Network

The feedforward neural networks with multiple layers have been widely used in practical applications. The network topology typically includes one input layer of sensory nodes, one or more hidden layers of computation nodes, and an output layer [13]. The neural activation and computation propagate through the forward pass, but the error correction follows the backward pass. Multilayer perceptron (MLP) and radial basis function network (RBFN) are two typical feedforward networks. The MLP that consists of several sigmoid nonlinear nodes in the hidden layers is commonly trained by the back-propagation algorithm or other optimization-based supervised learning methods. For a MLP, different weight initializations or configurations of network topologies (number of hidden nodes and hidden layers, activation functions, etc.) may result in different performance [43, 44]. Other than the MLP, the RBFN typically contains only one hidden layer, as shown in Fig. 4.1.

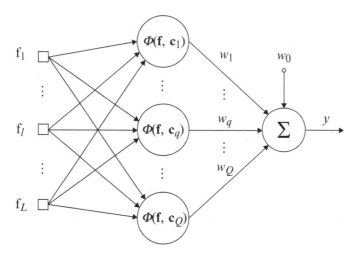

Fig. 4.1 The structure of a radial basis function network (RBFN)

The RBFN works by making a nonlinear transformation from the input space to a high-dimensional hidden space, and then produces responses through a linear output layer [13]. Park and Sandberg [27], and Hornik et al. [14] have justified in theory that any continuous function on a compact interval can be interpolated with arbitrary accuracy by a well-devised RBFN that contains a sufficiently large number of hidden neurons. Although there is not yet a rigorous theoretical framework that specifies the routine how to determine an optimal RBFN structure with the stated approximation properties, the RBFN has been extensively applied in analysis of VAG signal patterns [28, 30, 32].

Assume that the training data set consists of N signals, each of which is represented with the pairs of L-dimensional input features $\mathbf{f}^n = [f_1^n, f_2^n, \cdots f_L^n]^T$ and desired class label y_d^n, in the form of $\{\mathbf{f}^n, y_d^n\}_{n=1}^N$. The RBFN with Q hidden neurons produces the output response as

$$y^n = \sum_{q=1}^{Q} w_q \phi(\mathbf{f}^n, \mathbf{c}_q) + w_0, \tag{4.6}$$

where $\phi(\cdot)$ represents the radial basis kernel function, $\mathbf{c}_q$ is the center vector for the qth hidden node, w_q denotes the weight that connects the qth hidden node and the network output, and w_0 is the bias. The nonlinearity kernel $\phi(\cdot)$ can be the cubic function, thin-plate-spline function, multiquadratic function, or Gaussian function [13]. For the typical Gaussian function, the inner kernel $\phi(\mathbf{f}^n, \mathbf{c}_q)$ is then computed as

$$\phi(\mathbf{f}^n, \mathbf{c}_q) = \exp\left(-\left\|\mathbf{f}^n - \mathbf{c}_q\right\|^2 \Big/ \sigma^2\right), \tag{4.7}$$

where σ represents the spread parameter that determines the width of the area to which each hidden neuron responds.

The selection of radial basis function centers is a noteworthy factor that may affect the classification performance [28]. The centers of the RBFN are chosen from the training data set that contains total N signal instances. Selecting radial basis function centers in a random manner commonly leads to consumption of too many computational resources. The orthogonal least-squares method proposed by Chen et al. [3] can effectively select necessary centers that helps significantly reduce the computation costs for the RBFN. The aim of the orthogonal least-squares method is to perform a systematic selection of less than N centers so that the network complexity can be decreased with minimal degradation during the learning procedure [3]. At each regression step, a new center is selected in correspondence with the input features to maximize the variance increment of the desired output.

When Q $(Q < N)$ centers are selected, the orthogonal least-squares method treats the RBFN as a regression model, whose input-output mapping in Eq. (4.6) is expressed as [28]

$$\begin{bmatrix} y_d^1 \\ \vdots \\ y_d^n \\ \vdots \\ y_d^N \end{bmatrix} = \begin{bmatrix} 1 & \phi(\mathbf{f}^1, \mathbf{c}_1) & \cdots & \phi(\mathbf{f}^1, \mathbf{c}_Q) \\ \vdots & \vdots & \ddots & \vdots \\ 1 & \phi(\mathbf{f}^n, \mathbf{c}_1) & \cdots & \phi(\mathbf{f}^n, \mathbf{c}_Q) \\ \vdots & \vdots & \ddots & \vdots \\ 1 & \phi(\mathbf{f}^N, \mathbf{c}_1) & \cdots & \phi(\mathbf{f}^N, \mathbf{c}_Q) \end{bmatrix} \begin{bmatrix} w_0 \\ \vdots \\ w_q \\ \vdots \\ w_I \end{bmatrix} + \begin{bmatrix} \varepsilon^1 \\ \vdots \\ \varepsilon^n \\ \vdots \\ \varepsilon^N \end{bmatrix}, \qquad (4.8)$$

or written in compact the matrix form as

$$\mathbf{y}_d = \Phi \mathbf{w} + \varepsilon, \qquad (4.9)$$

where Φ is the N-by-$(Q+1)$ regression matrix with radial basis function centers, the weight vector $\mathbf{w} = [w_0, w_1, \cdots, w_Q]^T$, and ε represents the regression error vector term. The optimal weights obtained with the orthogonal least-squares method are given by

$$\mathbf{w}^* = (\Phi^T \Phi)^{-1} \Phi^T \mathbf{y}_d = \Phi^+ \mathbf{y}_d, \qquad (4.10)$$

where Φ^+ denotes the pseudoinverse of the regression matrix Φ. For a testing signal with input features $\mathbf{f}_t$, the RBFN provides the output response as

$$y_t = \Phi_t \mathbf{w}^* = \begin{bmatrix} 1, \phi_1, \phi_2, \ldots, \phi_Q \end{bmatrix} \mathbf{w}^*, \qquad (4.11)$$

where ϕ_q represents the radial basis function kernel $\phi(\mathbf{f}_t, \mathbf{c}_q)$.

4.4 Support Vector Machines

4.4.1 Vapnik Support Vector Machine

The support vector machine methodology proposed by Cortes and Vapnik [4] is based on the Vapnik-Chervonenkis dimension theory [38] and the structural risk minimization rule [37]. The support vector machine is a type of supervised learning paradigm that applies a nonlinear kernel mapping to project the training data onto a sufficiently higher dimension. A kernel function $\kappa(\cdot)$ is defined as the inner product of the nonlinear mapping operator $\varphi(\mathbf{f})$ as

$$\kappa(\mathbf{f}_j, \mathbf{f}_k) = \varphi(\mathbf{f}_j)^T \varphi(\mathbf{f}_k). \qquad (4.12)$$

By choosing appropriate nonlinear inner-product kernels, the SVM is able to perform the same function as the polynomial learning machine (with polynomial kernels), the radial basis function network (with Gaussian kernels), or the multilayer perceptron with a single hidden layer (with sigmoid kernels) [5].

Given a set of training data $\{\mathbf{f}_n, y_n\}$, with the class label $y_n \in \{-1, +1\}$, the SVM introduces a set of slack variables $\xi_n \geq 0$ to tolerate misclassification of nonseparable data in the mapped high-dimensional space. For a binary classification task, the boundaries of the margin can be expressed as

$$\begin{cases} \mathbf{w}^T \varphi(\mathbf{f}_n) + b \geq 1 - \xi_n, & \text{if } y_n = +1 \\ \mathbf{w}^T \varphi(\mathbf{f}_n) + b \leq -1 + \xi_n, & \text{if } y_n = -1 \end{cases} \qquad (4.13)$$

or written in a compact and equivalent inequality form as

$$y_n \left[\mathbf{w}^T \varphi(\mathbf{f}_n) + b \right] \geq 1 - \xi_n, \ n = 1, \cdots, N. \qquad (4.14)$$

If the training data mapped by kernel functions are linearly separable in the high-dimensional space, the slack variables $\xi_n = 0$.

Schematic representation of a typical support vector machine for pattern classifications is shown in Fig. 4.2. With the nonlinear kernel projections and slack variables, the SVM searches for the linear optimal decision hyperplane that maximizes the margin in the high-dimensional mapping space. The SVM selects a number of essential training data, which are considered to be the most informative

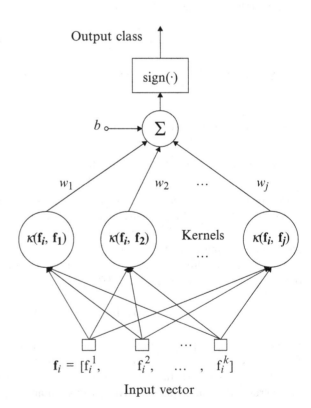

Fig. 4.2 Structure of a support vector machine (SVM) for pattern classifications (Adapted with permission from Ref. [42]. © 2011 Elsevier)

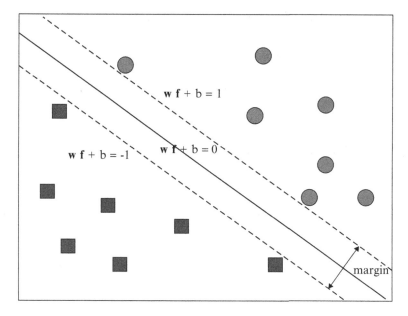

Fig. 4.3 Decision boundary margin of a support vector machine

for classifications, to outline the hyperplane boundaries of different classes. As shown in Fig. 4.3, the margin is defined as the distance between the hyperplane boundaries, which is equal to $2/(\mathbf{w}^T \mathbf{w})$. Because the maximization of the SVM margin also corresponds to minimizing its reciprocal $(\mathbf{w}^T \mathbf{w})/2$, the optimization problem of the SVM becomes

$$
\begin{cases}
\min\limits_{\mathbf{w}, \xi} & \frac{\mathbf{w}^T \mathbf{w}}{2} + C \sum\limits_{n=1}^{N} \xi_n \\
\text{s.t.} & y_n \left[\mathbf{w}^T \varphi(\mathbf{f}_n) + b \right] \geq 1 - \xi_n \\
& \xi_n \geq 0, \ n = 1, \cdots, N
\end{cases}
\tag{4.15}
$$

where C is a user-specified positive real constant that represents the penalty of misclassifying the training data. Based on the Lagrangian formulation, such a constrained quadratic problem can be written as

$$
L_{\mathrm{QP}} = \frac{\mathbf{w}^T \mathbf{w}}{2} + C \sum_{n=1}^{N} \xi_n - \sum_{n=1}^{N} \lambda_n \left\{ y_n [\mathbf{w}^T \varphi(\mathbf{f}_n) + b] - 1 + \xi_n \right\} - \sum_{n=1}^{N} \mu_n \xi_n,
\tag{4.16}
$$

with the nonnegative Lagrange multipliers $\lambda_n \geq 0$, $\mu_n \geq 0$, for $n = 1, \cdots, N$.

Setting the first-order derivative of L_{QP} with respect to $\mathbf{w}$, b, and ξ_n to zero yields

$$
\begin{cases}
\frac{\partial L_{QP}}{\partial \mathbf{w}} \Rightarrow & \mathbf{w} = \sum_{n=1}^{N} \lambda_n y_n \varphi(\mathbf{f}_n) \\
\frac{\partial L_{QP}}{\partial b} \Rightarrow & \sum_{n=1}^{N} \lambda_n y_n = 0 \\
\frac{\partial L_{QP}}{\partial \xi_n} \Rightarrow & C - \lambda_n - \mu_n = 0
\end{cases}
\tag{4.17}
$$

By substituting Eq. (4.17) into Eq. (4.16), one can obtain the dual Lagrangian problem

$$
L_{DP} = \frac{1}{2} \sum_{j=1}^{N} \sum_{k=1}^{N} y_j y_k \kappa(\mathbf{f}_j, \mathbf{f}_k) \lambda_j \lambda_k + C \sum_{j=1}^{N} \xi_j
\tag{4.18}
$$

$$
- \sum_{j=1}^{N} \lambda_j \left\{ y_j \left[\sum_{k=1}^{N} \lambda_j y_k \kappa(\mathbf{f}_j, \mathbf{f}_k) + b \right] - 1 + \xi_j \right\} - \sum_{j=1}^{N} (C - \lambda_j) \xi_j
$$

$$
= \sum_{i=1}^{N} \lambda_i - \frac{1}{2} \sum_{j=1}^{N} \sum_{k=1}^{N} y_j y_k \kappa(\mathbf{f}_j, \mathbf{f}_k) \lambda_j \lambda_k.
$$

To solve such a dual problem, we may consider the Karush-Kuhn-Tucker (KKT) conditions to transform the inequality constrains into the equality constrains as

$$
\begin{cases}
\lambda_j \left\{ y_j [\mathbf{w}^T \varphi(\mathbf{f}_j) + b] - 1 + \xi_j \right\} = 0 \\
\mu_j \xi_j = 0 \\
\xi_j \geq 0, \ \lambda_j \geq 0, \ \mu_j \geq 0
\end{cases}
\tag{4.19}
$$

From $\mu_j \xi_j = 0$, we may select two elements $\xi_j^* = 0$ and $\lambda_j^* > 0$ from the solution $(\mathbf{w}^*, \xi^*, \lambda^*, \mu^*)$ to compute the bias term as

$$
b = 1/y_j - \mathbf{w}^T \varphi(\mathbf{f}_j),
\tag{4.20}
$$

in which the data point $\{\mathbf{f}_j, y_j\}$ may be picked up from the training data for which $\lambda_j^* > 0$. Therefore, the SVM performs the nonlinear pattern classification as below

$$
y_j = y_j(\mathbf{f}_j) = \text{sign} \left[\sum_{k=1}^{N} \lambda_k y_k \kappa(\mathbf{f}_j, \mathbf{f}_k) + b \right].
\tag{4.21}
$$

4.4.2 Least-Squares Support Vector Machine

The least-squares support vector machine (LS-SVM) was proposed by Suykens et al. [34], with the basic concept of modifying the Vapnik SVM classification network to become the regularized regression network with a squared loss function. The LS-SVM treats the class label y_n as a real target value instead of a binary threshold. Misclassifications could be tolerated in the case of overlapping distributions with a target value error variable [34]. Then, a squared loss function is used to simplify the primal SVM problem. Such modifications allows the LS-SVM to solve the dual problem more easily than solving a set of linear equations. Compared with the Vapnik SVM, the LS-SVM has an improvement of moderate complexity and works more efficiently, which is the reason that we considered the LS-SVM instead of the Vapnik SVM in the present study. The major differences between the Vapnik SVM and the LS-SVM are summarized as follows [34]:

- The optimization of the Vapnik SVM is obtained by solving a constrained quadratic programming problem related to the convex cost function, whereas the LS-SVM reformulates the convex cost function to be a regularized function in the squared sense. The optimization of the LS-SVM is achieved by solving a set of linear KKT equations. Therefore, compared with the Vapnik SVM, the LS-SVM has a modest computation complexity which leads to higher performance.
- The solution vector of Lagrange multipliers obtained by the Vapnik SVM is sparse, i.e., only the Lagrange multipliers assigned to the representative training data points (support vectors) are with non-zero values, and the values of the rest Lagrange multipliers (for the remaining subset of training data) are equal to zero. For the LS-SVM, on the other hand, all the training data contribute to the model, because no Lagrange multiplier will be exactly equal to zero. Or in other words, every training data point is a support vector to contribute in the classification decision making. Nevertheless, Suykens et al. [34] pointed out that, after optimizing the LS-SVM, the Lagrange multipliers assigned to the representative data points in the training set are with large absolute values, and the others for those less important training data have small absolute values (or close to zero). In other words, although the solution of Lagrange multipliers provided by the LS-SVM is not sparse, the support vectors can still be picked up from the optimum solution by defining a threshold level (Table 4.1).

4.5 Bayesian Decision Rule

Bayesian decision rule is based on Bayesian interpretation of conditional probability, which infers a posterior probability with the prior probability, class-conditional probability, and evidence. According to Bayes' formula, the joint probability density

Table 4.1 A optimization paradigm of the least squares support vector machine (Adapted with permission from Ref. [42]. © 2011 Elsevier)

Training set: $\{\mathbf{f}_i, y_i\}_{i=1}^N$;

features of the ith input pattern: $\mathbf{f}_i$;

class label: $y_i \in \{-1, 1\}$ (negative or positive);

Classification: $y_i = y(\mathbf{f}_i) = \mathrm{sign}[\mathbf{w}^T \varphi(\mathbf{f}_i) + b]$, where $\varphi(\cdot)$ represents the high-dimensional mapping in feature space, and c denotes the bias;

Optimization problem:

$$
\begin{cases}
\min\limits_{\mathbf{w},c,e}\ J(\mathbf{w}, \mathbf{e}) = \frac{1}{2}\mathbf{w}^T\mathbf{w} + \gamma \sum\limits_{i=1}^N e_i^2 \\
\text{s.t.}\ \ y_i[\mathbf{w}^T\varphi(\mathbf{f}_i) + b] = 1 - e_i,
\end{cases}
$$

where γ is the regularization parameter that controls the tradeoff between the complexity of the machine and the number of nonseparable data points, and e_i represent error variables that measure the deviation of a data point from the ideal condition of pattern separability;

Lagrangian:

$$
L(\mathbf{w}, b, \mathbf{e}; \alpha) = J(\mathbf{w}, \mathbf{e}) - \sum_{i=1}^N \alpha_i \left\{ y_i[\mathbf{w}^T\varphi(\mathbf{f}_i) + b] - 1 + e_i \right\};
$$

Lagrange multiples: $\alpha = [\alpha_1, \cdots, \alpha_N]^T$;

Conditions for optimality:

$$
\begin{cases}
\frac{\partial L}{\partial \mathbf{w}} = 0 \rightarrow \mathbf{w} = \sum\limits_{i=1}^N \alpha_i y_i \varphi(\mathbf{f}_i) \\
\frac{\partial L}{\partial b} = 0 \rightarrow \sum\limits_{i=1}^N \alpha_i y_i = 0 \\
\frac{\partial L}{\partial e_i} = 0 \rightarrow \alpha_i = \gamma e_i,\ i = 1, \cdots, N \\
\frac{\partial L}{\partial \alpha_i} = 0 \rightarrow y_i[\mathbf{w}^T\varphi(\mathbf{f}_i) + b] - 1 + e_i = 0,\ i = 1, \cdots, N
\end{cases}
$$

The equivalent linear system:

$$
\begin{bmatrix}
\mathbf{I} & 0 & 0 & -\mathbf{Z}^T \\
0 & 0 & 0 & -\mathbf{Y}^T \\
0 & 0 & \gamma\mathbf{I} & -\mathbf{I} \\
\mathbf{Z} & \mathbf{Y} & \mathbf{I} & 0
\end{bmatrix}
\begin{bmatrix}
\mathbf{w} \\ b \\ \mathbf{e} \\ \alpha
\end{bmatrix}
=
\begin{bmatrix}
0 \\ 0 \\ 0 \\ \mathbf{I}_v
\end{bmatrix},
$$

where $\mathbf{Z} = [\varphi(\mathbf{f}_1)^T y_1, \cdots, \varphi(\mathbf{f}_N)^T y_N]^T$, $\mathbf{Y} = [y_1, \cdots, y_N]^T$, $\mathbf{I}$ is a unit matrix, $\mathbf{I}_v = [1, \cdots, 1]^T$,

$\mathbf{e} = [e_1, \cdots, e_N]^T, \alpha = [\alpha_1, \cdots, \alpha_N]^T$;

Elimination of $\mathbf{w}$ and $\mathbf{e}$ gives:

$$
\begin{bmatrix}
0 & \mathbf{Y}^T \\
\mathbf{Y} & \mathbf{Z}^T\mathbf{Z} + \mathbf{I}/\gamma
\end{bmatrix}
\begin{bmatrix}
b \\ \alpha
\end{bmatrix}
=
\begin{bmatrix}
0 \\ \mathbf{I}_v
\end{bmatrix};
$$

The kernel trick is applied to the matrix $\Omega = \mathbf{Z}^T\mathbf{Z}$,

with $\Omega_{ij} = y_i y_j \varphi(\mathbf{f}_i)^T \varphi(\mathbf{f}_j) = y_i y_j \kappa(\mathbf{f}_i, \mathbf{f}_j)$, $i, j = 1, \cdots, N$;

The corresponding LS-SVM classification in the dual space:

$$
y_i = y(\mathbf{f}_i) = \mathrm{sign}\left[\sum_{j=1}^N \alpha_j y_j \kappa(\mathbf{f}_i, \mathbf{f}_j) + b \right];
$$

α_j are also used to determine the support vectors;

of a signal with input feature vector $\mathbf{f}$ belonging to a particular group ω, $\omega \in \{\omega_N, \omega_A\}$, can be written as [45, 47]

$$p(\mathbf{f}, \omega) = p(\mathbf{f}|\omega)P(\omega) = P(\omega|\mathbf{f})p(\mathbf{f}), \tag{4.22}$$

where $P(\omega)$ is the prior probability that indicates the occurrence of a signal group (healthy normal group: ω_N or pathological abnormal group: ω_A), $P(\omega|\mathbf{f})$ is the posterior probability that describes the probability of the state of a signal being in the group ω with respect to the corresponding measured feature vector $\mathbf{f}$. For the VAG signal classification, the evidence factor $p(\mathbf{f})$ is the sum of the product between the class-conditional probability density and prior probability for the normal and abnormal signal groups, i.e.,

$$p(\mathbf{f}) = p(\mathbf{f}|\omega_N)P(\omega_N) + p(\mathbf{f}|\omega_A)P(\omega_A). \tag{4.23}$$

Therefore, the posterior probability $P(\omega|\mathbf{f})$ can be computed as [5]:

$$P(\omega|\mathbf{f}) = \frac{p(\mathbf{f}|\omega)P(\omega)}{p(\mathbf{f}|\omega_N)P(\omega_N) + p(\mathbf{f}|\omega_A)P(\omega_A)}. \tag{4.24}$$

With the measured feature vector $\mathbf{f}$, the classifier makes the decision by assigning the class label to a given VAG signal based on the maximal posterior probability criterion as

$$\underset{\omega \in \omega_N, \omega_A}{\arg\max} P(\omega|\mathbf{f}). \tag{4.25}$$

4.6   Multiple Classifier System

In addition to single classifiers, the multiple classifier system methodology would be an excellent option to improve diagnostic performance. When dealing a data set with finite size and noisy instances, different classifiers may exhibit diverse generalization abilities and provide various decision boundaries. Some classifiers may be good at making wonderful local decisions in particular regions, but could have some defects for the global generalization.

As a recent emerging machine learning methodology based on the principle of "divide and conquer" [13], classifier combination was widely used by researchers [11, 12, 17, 19, 35], with the purpose of achieving better performance over an individual classifier. By combing a finite number of component neural networks (CNNs) with a well-devised combination rule [12, 17, 35] or fusion strategy [19, 44], a neural network ensemble is expected to provide an informative overall decision that is supposedly superior to that attained by any one of the CNNs acting solely [13].

The most popular ensemble algorithms are AdaBoost [9] and Bagging [1]. The AdaBoost works by repeatedly training a given type of weak-learning machine from different distributed training data sets, and then combining their outputs. The distribution of the training data for the current CNN is boosted depending on the performance of previous CNNs, i.e., the training data that are incorrectly predicted by previous CNNs will be chosen with priority to the training of the current CNN. In spite of the effectiveness, the AdaBoost is very sensitive to outliers and sometimes results in overfitting [33]. On the other hand, the Bagging algorithm introduces the bootstrap approach [6] into the training data resampling procedure [1], and aggregates the CNNs with the simple average strategy [13]. In the bootstrap procedure, each data sample is selected separately at random from the original data set such that a particular data sample could appear multiple times in a bootstrap-generated data set. The bias of the Bagging ensemble would converge by averaging while the variance falls much smaller than that of each CNN.

Since the LS-SVM is not a weak-learning machine [34], we use the Bagging algorithm rather than the AdaBoost for the ensemble of five component LS-SVMs (CSVMs) which are labeled from CSVM1 to CSVM5 in numerical sequence. The CSVMs combined with the Bagging algorithm are trained by different bootstrap-generated data sets. The number of signals in each bootstrap-generated data set is of equal size to the original VAG data set. The testing data set for each CSVM is the same as the original VAG data set. Because the training data for each CSVM are generated using the bootstrap approach, it is not necessary to apply the LOO method to the ensemble system any more.

According to the linear combination rule of the Bagging, the CSVMs are simply averaged in the ensemble, so that the effectiveness of the ensemble would be affected by some of the CSVMs with poor performance, because the simple average strategy treats all the CSVMs equally. In order to utilize the diverse knowledge generated by the CSVMs, we use a dynamic weighted fusion (DWF) rule that can adaptively combine the CSVMs in the classifier fusion system [2, 40].

Suppose that a total of K CSVMs are linearly combined in the classifier fusion system. The local decision generated by the kth CSVM is denoted as $g_k(\mathbf{f}^n)$, with regards to the feature vector of the nth VAG signal, $\mathbf{f}^n$. The classifier fusion system then provides the overall classification decision, $g_{DWF}(\mathbf{f}^n)$, by linearly combining the CSVMs with the weights $w_k(\mathbf{f}^n)$ that are varied from one signal to another [2]. Thus the DWF-based ensemble output can be formulated as [2]

$$g_{DWF}(\mathbf{f}^n) = \sum_{k=1}^{K} w_k(\mathbf{f}^n) g_k(\mathbf{f}^n). \tag{4.26}$$

And the nonnegative and normalization constraints on the weights, as widely accepted in the literature [12, 35, 44], can be written as

$$\sum_{k=1}^{K} w_k(\mathbf{f}^n) = 1, \; w_k(\mathbf{f}^n) \geq 0. \tag{4.27}$$

The task of the DWF is to determine the fusion weights that help the ensemble system provide an overall classification decision with higher accuracy. To achieve this goal, let us study the error term of the CSVMs and the DWF-based ensemble. Concerning the kth CSVM, the squared error that characterizes the difference between the local decision and the desired class label, $l(\mathbf{f}^n)$, in relation to the nth VAG signal is

$$e_k^2(\mathbf{f}^n) = [l(\mathbf{f}^n) - g_k(\mathbf{f}^n)]^2. \tag{4.28}$$

Then, the squared error of the ensemble, $e_{DWF}^2(\mathbf{f}^n)$, is estimated in an analogous manner to that of each CSVM. Consider that the fusion weights are normalized, as presented in Eq. (4.27), the class label $l(\mathbf{f}^n)$ can be split by multiplying the fusion weights, so that $e_{DWF}^2(\mathbf{f}^n)$ is derived as follows:

$$
\begin{aligned}
e_{DWF}^2(\mathbf{f}^n) &= \left[l(\mathbf{f}^n) - \sum_{k=1}^{K} w_k(\mathbf{f}^n) g_k(\mathbf{f}^n) \right]^2 \\
&= \left[\sum_{k=1}^{K} w_k(\mathbf{f}^n) l(\mathbf{f}^n) - \sum_{k=1}^{K} w_k(\mathbf{f}^n) g_k(\mathbf{f}^n) \right]^2 \\
&= \left\{ \sum_{k=1}^{K} w_k(\mathbf{f}^n) \left[l(\mathbf{f}^n) - g_k(\mathbf{f}^n) \right] \right\} \left\{ \sum_{j=1}^{K} w_j(\mathbf{f}^n) \left[l(\mathbf{f}^n) - g_j(\mathbf{f}^n) \right] \right\} \\
&= \sum_{k=1}^{K} \sum_{j=1}^{K} w_k(\mathbf{f}^n) w_j(\mathbf{f}^n) \left[l(\mathbf{f}^n) - g_k(\mathbf{f}^n) \right] \left[l(\mathbf{f}^n) - g_j(\mathbf{f}^n) \right] \\
&= \sum_{k=1}^{K} \sum_{j=1}^{K} w_k(\mathbf{f}^n) w_j(\mathbf{f}^n) e_k(\mathbf{f}^n) e_j(\mathbf{f}^n), \tag{4.29}
\end{aligned}
$$

where $e_k(\mathbf{f}^n) = [l(\mathbf{f}^n) - g_k(\mathbf{f}^n)]$ represents the instantaneous error of the kth CSVM.

Considering Eqs. (4.27) and (4.29), the minimization of the squared error of the ensemble is equivalent to the constrained quadratic programming (CQP) problem specified below:

$$
\begin{cases}
\text{minimize} \quad e_{DWF}^2(\mathbf{f}^n) = \sum_{k=1}^{K} \sum_{j=1}^{K} w_k(\mathbf{f}^n) w_j(\mathbf{f}^n) e_k(\mathbf{f}^n) e_j(\mathbf{f}^n), \\
\text{subject to} \quad \sum_{k=1}^{K} w_k(\mathbf{f}^n) = 1, \ w_k(\mathbf{f}^n) \geq 0.
\end{cases} \tag{4.30}
$$

In order to solve the CQP problem presented in Eq. (4.30), we apply the Lagrange multiplier method [26] and define the cost function as

$$C(w_1(\mathbf{f}^n), \cdots, w_K(\mathbf{f}^n), \lambda(\mathbf{f}^n))$$

$$= \sum_{k=1}^{K} \sum_{j=1}^{K} w_k(\mathbf{f}^n) w_j(\mathbf{f}^n) e_k(\mathbf{f}^n) e_j(\mathbf{f}^n) - \lambda(\mathbf{f}^n) \left[\sum_{k=1}^{K} w_k(\mathbf{f}^n) - 1 \right], \quad (4.31)$$

where the nonnegative coefficient $\lambda(\mathbf{f}^n)$ represents the Lagrange multiplier, which varies from one signal to another.

According to the weak Lagrangian principle [26], the optimum solution to the CQP problem, $\{\mathbf{w}^*(\mathbf{f}^n), \lambda^*(\mathbf{f}^n)\}$, is the stationary point of the cost function presented in Eq. (4.31), and satisfies the following unique equations:

$$\begin{cases} \frac{\partial C(w_1(\mathbf{f}^n), \cdots, w_K(\mathbf{f}^n), \lambda(\mathbf{f}^n))}{\partial w_k(\mathbf{f}^n)} = 2 \sum_{j=1}^{K} w_j(\mathbf{f}^n) e_k(\mathbf{f}^n) e_j(\mathbf{f}^n) - \lambda(\mathbf{f}^n) = 0, \\ \frac{\partial C(w_1(\mathbf{f}^n), \cdots, w_K(\mathbf{f}^n), \lambda(\mathbf{f}^n))}{\partial \lambda(\mathbf{f}^n)} = \sum_{k=1}^{K} w_k(\mathbf{f}^n) - 1 = 0. \end{cases} \quad (4.32)$$

The optimal weights $w_k(\mathbf{f}^n)$ of the DWF that minimize the squared error of the ensemble system can be obtained by solving Eq. (4.32), i.e.,

$$w_k^*(\mathbf{f}^i) = \frac{\sum_{j=1}^{K} e_k^{-1}(\mathbf{f}^n) e_j^{-1}(\mathbf{f}^n)}{\sum_{i=1}^{K} \sum_{j=1}^{K} e_i^{-1}(\mathbf{f}^n) e_j^{-1}(\mathbf{f}^n)}, \quad k = 1, \cdots, K. \quad (4.33)$$

Because the error term of the CSVM can be estimated when the nth VAG class label $l(\mathbf{f}^n)$ is given and the CSVM model parameters are specified, the optimal fusion weights can be directly computed according to Eq. (4.33).

Now let us divert our attention to the DWF-based ensemble error term. Considering Eqs. (4.29) and (4.33), we have

$$e_{DWF}^2(\mathbf{f}^n) = \sum_{k=1}^{K} \sum_{j=1}^{K} w_k(\mathbf{f}^n) w_j(\mathbf{f}^n) e_k(\mathbf{f}^n) e_j(\mathbf{f}^n)$$

$$= \frac{1}{\sum_{i=1}^{K} \sum_{j=1}^{K} e_i^{-1}(\mathbf{f}^n) e_j^{-1}(\mathbf{f}^n)}. \quad (4.34)$$

It is clear that both of $e_k^2(\mathbf{f}^n)$ and $e_{DWF}^2(\mathbf{f}^n)$ are nonnegative, i.e., $e_k^2(\mathbf{f}^n) \geq 0$ and $\sum_{i=1}^{K} \sum_{j=1}^{K} e_i^{-1}(\mathbf{f}^n) e_j^{-1}(\mathbf{f}^n) \geq 0$. To compare with the squared error of the CSVM, we may employ the division operator such that

$$\frac{e_k^2(\mathbf{f}^n)}{e_{DWF}^2(\mathbf{f}^n)} = 1 + \sum_{\substack{i=1 \\ i \neq k}}^{K} \sum_{\substack{j=1 \\ j \neq k}}^{K} \frac{e_k^2(\mathbf{f}^n)}{e_i(\mathbf{f}^n)e_j(\mathbf{f}^n)} \geq 1. \tag{4.35}$$

Therefore the optimal fusion weights derived in Eq. (4.35) guarantee that the DWF-based ensemble system more or less likely outperforms a single CSVM.

4.7 Classification Performance Evaluations

As we know, the classification performance depends on a vast variety of factors, such as classifier design, input features, model validation methods, and so forth. The cross-validation method is most frequently used to validate the generalization ability of a classifier model. In the L-fold cross-validation experiments, the available data set is randomly divided into L disjoint subsets. The L-1 subsets are used for training, and the remaining subset is used for testing. Then, the procedure is repeated for L trials, each time using a different subset for validation. For a data set of N instances, if the fold number L equals $N/2$, such a scheme is called hold-out cross-validation (50 % of the data instances for training and the resting 50 % instances holding out for testing). If the fold number L is equal to N, which indicates leaving every single instance for testing and all the other instances for training, such a validation scheme is named as leave-one-out (LOO) cross-validation.

The confusion matrix is a contingency table that is commonly used to interpret the classification results. For a binary classification task, the confusion matrix is defined in Table 4.2. According to the confusion matrix, we may compute the following parameters:

$$\text{Sensitivity (True Positive Rate)} = \frac{TP}{TP + FN} \tag{4.36}$$

$$\text{Specificity (True Negative Rate)} = \frac{TN}{FP + TN} \tag{4.37}$$

$$\text{Precision (Positive Predictive Value)} = \frac{TP}{TP + FP} \tag{4.38}$$

$$\text{Overall Accuracy} = \frac{TP + TN}{TP + FP + FN + TN} \tag{4.39}$$

Table 4.2 The diagnostic confusion matrix for classification performance evaluation

	Actual positives	Actual negatives
Classified positives	True positive (TP)	False positive (FP)
Classified negatives	False negative (FN)	True negative (TN)

A receiver operating characteristic (ROC) curve is a graphical tool for binary classification performance evaluation [22]. The curve is established by computing the fraction of true positive rate over the fraction of false positive rate at different threshold levels. The area under the ROC curve (AUC or A_z) is referred to as the probability that a classifier will rank a randomly chosen positive instance higher than a randomly chosen negative one according to a threshold parameter [7]. The value of AUC is frequently used to evaluate the discrimination capability of a classifier. A random binary classification produces an AUC value of 0.5, and a perfect sensitivity classification corresponds the AUC value equal to 1.

4.8 VAG Signal Classification Results Comparison

In this section, we will review the knee joint VAG signal classification results reported in the recent literature. Moussavi et al. [24] applied the forward-backward linear prediction (FBLP) model to generate the variance of means (VM), 40 FBLP model coefficients, and 10 dominant poles of FBLP model features from VAG signal segments. They combined these FBLP features and the clinical parameters (ausculation sound, activity level, and age) and used the logistic regression analysis method to screen the signal segments. Their results showed that the logistic regression analysis method trained by 262 signal segments can recognize 184 segments from 239 testing VAG segments (accuracy: 77 %, sensitivity: 0.7259, specificity: 0.8269). The early work of Rangayyan et al. [31] reported that the logistic regression analysis classifier, input with features of autoregressive coefficients, cepstral coefficients, and dominant poles, was able to provide an overall classification rate of 75.6 %.

Table 4.3 summarizes the diagnostic results reported by the recent studies in the last decade [2, 18, 25, 28–30, 32, 36, 41, 45]. Krishnan et al. [18] computed the optimal matching pursuit time-frequency distribution (TFD) of VAG signals. They considered the mean of energy parameter (EP), energy spread parameter (ESP), standard deviation of frequency parameter (FP), standard deviation of frequency spread parameter (FSP), and coefficients of variations of EP and ESP, as the dominant features. The logistic regression analysis technique was employed to perform the signal classifications (accuracy: 68.9 %, sensitivity: 0.56, specificity: 0.78) [18]. Kim et al. [16] extracted the EP, ESP, FP, FSP features from the enhanced TFD of VAG signal segments, and then used a back-propagation neural network to implement pattern classifications (accuracy: 95.4 %, sensitivity: 0.92, specificity: 0.9868). Umapathy et al. [36] used to Daubechies db4 wavelets constructe the local discriminant base (LDB) tree to measure the dissimilarity between the wavelet basis coefficients. The linear discriminant analysis (LDA) provided an overall accuracy of 76.4 % with sensitivity of 0.7895. Rangayyan and Wu [28] extracted the form factor (FF), skewness (S), kurtosis (K), and Shannon entropy (H) features to describe the variability in VAG signals. Based on these four variability features, the radial basis function network (RBFN) [28] and strict 2-surface proximal classifier [25] provided the overall accuracy of 82.02 % (sensitivity: 0.7105 and specificity: 0.902)

Table 4.3 The diagnostic results of different classification methods with the knee joint vibroarthrographic signal features developed in the previous studies [2, 18, 25, 28–30, 32, 36, 41, 45, 46]

Feature sets	Classification methods	Evaluation	Accuracy (%)	Sensitivity	Specificity	A_z
EP, ESP, FP, FSP CV1, CV2	Logistic regression analysis [18]	LOO	68.9	0.5641	0.7843	N/A
MLDB nodes	Linear discriminant analysis [36]	LOO	76.4	0.7895	0.7451	N/A
FF, S, K, H	Radial basis function network [28]	LOO	82.02	0.7105	0.902	0.82
FF, S, K, H	Strict 2-surface proximal classifier [25]	LOO	91.01	0.9474	0.8824	0.95
EP, ESP, FP, FSP	Back-propagation neural network [16]	ATAT	95.4	0.92	0.9868	N/A
TC1, TC2, VMS1, VMS2	Radial basis function network [29]	LOO	89.89	0.9211	0.8824	0.9174
dKLD, K, H, μ, σ	Radial basis function network [30]	LOO	77.53	0.7105	0.8235	0.8322
FF, VMS	Bayesian decision rule [45]	LOO	86.67	0.75	0.9362	0.9096
FF, S, K, H, TC, VMS	Multiple classifier fusion system [41]	LOO	80.9	0.8947	0.9216	0.9484
Natom, TCFT	Dynamic weighted classifier fusion system [2]	LOO	88.76	0.7368	1	0.9515
FSI, AEA	Bayesian decision rule [46]	LOO	88	0.7143	0.9787	0.957
FF, dKLD, TC, FD, S	Radial basis function network [32]	LOO	100	1	1	0.961

MLDB modified local discriminant bases with db4 wavelet, *EP* mean energy parameter, *ESP* energy spread parameter, *FP* frequency parameter, *FSP* frequency spread parameter, *CV1* coefficient of variation of EP, *CV2* coefficient of variation of ESP, *FF* form factor, *S* skewness, *K* Kurtosis, *H* entropy, *TC* turns count, *TC1* turns count during knee extension, *TC2* turns count during knee flexion, *VMS* variance of mean-squared values, *VMS1* variance of mean-squared values during knee extension, *VMS2* variance of mean-squared values during knee flexion, *FSI* fractal scaling index, *AEA* averaged envelope amplitude, *dKLD* difference between the Kullback-Leibler distances of the normal and abnormal signal probability density functions, μ mean, σ, standard deviation, *FD* fractal dimensions, *Natom* number of wavelet matching pursuit decomposition, *TCFT* turns count with the fixed threshold, *LOO* leave-one-out method, *ATAT* all training all testing, *N/A* no applicable and 91.01 % (sensitivity: 0.9474 and specificity: 0.8824), respectively. Rangayyan and Wu then developed the temporal fluctuation features in terms of turns count (TC) and variance of mean-squared (VMS) values [29], and the difference between the Kullback-Leibler distances (dKLD) and other statistical parameters based on the signal probability density function (PDF) [30]. The RBFN classifier evaluated by the leave-one-out (LOO) method can produce the overall accuracy as high as 89.89 % (sensitivity: 0.92 and specificity: 0.88) and the area of 0.9174 under the ROC curve [29]. Some other computational methods such as k-nearest neighbor classifier ($k = 5$) [20], Bayesian decision rule [45], and the multiple classifier fusion system optimized by a recurrent neural network [41] were also applied to perform signal pattern classifications. The multiple classifier fusion system input with the combination of FF, S, K, H, TC, and VMS features may provide a slight improvement of area value 0.9484 under the ROC curve [41]. Yang et al. [46] extracted the features of fractal scaling index and averaged envelope amplitude to describe the subtle fluctuations in VAG signals. The classification results of the Bayesian decision rule based on these two fluctuation features (accuracy: 88 %, A_z: 0.957) [46] were better than the same classifier with the input features of FF and VMS (accuracy: 86.67 %, A_z: 0.9096) [45]. To improve the classification performance, Cai et al. [2] proposed the dynamic weighted classifier fusion system to distinguish VAG signals. The dynamic weighted classifier fusion system only with the number of wavelet matching pursuit decomposition and turns count with the fixed threshold as the input features was able to provide an overall accuracy of 88.76 % and the A_z value of 0.9515 under the ROC curve [2]. A combination of most informative features can also help a classifier improve the diagnostic performance. Rangayyan et al. [32] used the combination of FF, dKLD, TC, FD, and S features to train the radial basis function network, and produced the A_z value of 0.961 under the ROC curve [32].

References

1. Breiman L (1996) Bagging predictors. Mach Learn 24(2):123–140
2. Cai S, Yang S, Zheng F, Lu M, Wu Y, Krishnan S (2013) Knee joint vibration signal analysis with matching pursuit decomposition and dynamic weighted classifier fusion. Comput Math Methods Med 2013:Article ID 904267
3. Chen S, Cowan CFN, Grant PM (1991) Orthogonal least squares learning algorithm for radial basis function networks. IEEE Trans Neural Netw 2(2):302–309
4. Cortes C, Vapnik VN (1995) Support-vector networks. Mach Learn 20(3):273–297
5. Duda RO, Hart PE, Stork DG (2001) Pattern classification, 2nd edn. Wiley, New York
6. Efron B, Tibshirani R (1993) An introduction to the bootstrap. Chapman and Hall, New York
7. Fawcett T (2006) An introduction to ROC analysis. Pattern Recognit Lett 27(8):861–874
8. Fisher RA (1936) The use of multiple measurements in taxonomic problems. Ann Eugen 7(2):179–188
9. Freund Y, Schapire RE (1997) A decision-theoretic generalization of on-line learning and an application to boosting. J Comput Syst Sci 55(1):119–139

10. Guyon I, Elisseeff A (2003) An introduction to variable and feature selection. J Mach Learn Res 3:1157–1182
11. Hansen LK, Salamon P (1990) Neural network ensembles. IEEE Trans Pattern Anal Mach Intell 12(10):993–1001
12. Hashem S, Schmeiser B (1995) Improving model accuracy using optimal linear combinations of trained neural networks. IEEE Trans Neural Netw 6(3):792–794
13. Haykin S (1998) Neural networks: a comprehensive foundation, 2nd edn. Prentice Hall PTR, Englewood Cliffs
14. Hornik KM, Stinchcombe M, White H (1989) Multilayer feedforward networks are universal approximators. Neural Netw 2(5):359–366
15. Jain AK, Duin RPW, Mao JC (2000) Statistical pattern recognition: a review. IEEE Trans Pattern Anal Mach Intell 22(1):4–37
16. Kim KS, Seo JH, Kang JU, Song CG (2009) An enhanced algorithm for knee joint sound classification using feature extraction based on time-frequency analysis. Comput Methods Programs Biomed 94(2):198–206
17. Kittler J, Hatef M, Duin RPW, Matus J (1998) On combining classifiers. IEEE Trans Pattern Anal Mach Intell 20(3):226–239
18. Krishnan S, Rangayyan RM, Bell GD, Frank CB (2000) Adaptive time-frequency analysis of knee joint vibroarthrographic signals for noninvasive screening of articular cartilage pathology. IEEE Trans Biomed Eng 47(6):773–783
19. Kuncheva LI (2002) A theoretical study on six classifier fusion strategies. IEEE Trans Pattern Anal Mach Intell 24(2):281–286
20. Liu K, Luo X, Zheng F, Yang S, Cai S, Wu Y (2014) Classification of knee joint vibroarthrographic signals using k-nearest neighbor algorithm. In: Proceedings of the 27th Canadian conference on electrical and computer engineering, Toronto, pp 150–153
21. Marill T, Green DM (1963) On the effectiveness of receptors in recognition systems. IEEE Trans Inf Theory 9(1):11–17
22. Marques de Sa JP (2003) Applied statistics using SPSS, STATISTICA, and MATLAB. Springer, Berlin
23. Martinez AM, Kak AC (2001) PCA versus LDA. IEEE Trans Pattern Anal Mach Intell 23(2):228–233
24. Moussavi ZMK, Rangayyan RM, Bell GD, Frank CB, Ladly KO, Zhang YT (1996) Screening of vibroarthrographic signals via adaptive segmentation and linear prediction modeling. IEEE Trans Biomed Eng 43(1):15–23
25. Mu T, Nandi AK, Rangayyan RM (2008) Screening of knee-joint vibroarthrographic signals using the strict 2-surface proximal classifier and genetic algorithm. Comput Biol Med 38(10):1103–1111
26. Nash SG, Sofer A (1995) Linear and nonlinear programming. McGraw-Hill, Columbus
27. Park J, Sandberg IW (1991) Universal approximation using radial-basis-function networks. Neural Comput 3(2):246–257
28. Rangayyan RM, Wu YF (2008) Screening of knee-joint vibroarthrographic signals using statistical parameters and radial basis functions. Med Biol Eng Comput 46(3):223–232
29. Rangayyan RM, Wu Y (2009) Analysis of vibroarthrographic signals with features related to signal variability and radial-basis functions. Ann Biomed Eng 37(1):156–163
30. Rangayyan RM, Wu Y (2010) Screening of knee-joint vibroarthrographic signals using probability density functions estimated with Parzen windows. Biomed Signal Process Control 5(1):53–58
31. Rangayyan RM, Krishnan S, Bell GD, Frank CB, Ladly KO (1997) Parametric representation and screening of knee joint vibroarthrographic signals. IEEE Trans Biomed Eng 44(11):1068–1074
32. Rangayyan RM, Oloumi F, Wu Y, Cai S (2013) Fractal analysis of knee-joint vibroarthrographic signals via power spectral analysis. Biomed Signal Process Control 8(1):26–29
33. Ridgeway G (1999) The state of boosting. Comput Sci Stat 31:172–181

34. Suykens JAK, Van Gestel T, De Brabanter J, De Moor B, Vandewalle J (2002) Least squares support vector machines. World Scientific, Singapore
35. Ueda N (2000) Optimal linear combination of neural networks for improving classification performance. IEEE Trans Pattern Anal Mach Intell 22(2):207–215
36. Umapathy K, Krishnan S (2006) Modified local discriminant bases algorithm and its application in analysis of human knee joint vibration signals. IEEE Trans Biomed Eng 53(3):517–523
37. Vapnik VN (1998) Statistical learning theory. Wiley, New York
38. Vapnik VN, Chervonenkis AY (1971) On the uniform convergence of relative frequencies of events to their probabilities. Theory Probab Appl 16(2):264–280
39. Whitney AW (1971) A direct method of nonparametric measurement selection. IEEE Trans Comput 20(9):1100–1103
40. Wu Y, Krishnan S (2009) An adaptive classifier fusion method for analysis of knee-joint vibroarthrographic signals. In: Proceedings of 2009 international conference on computational intelligence for measurement systems and applications, Hong Kong, pp 190–193
41. Wu Y, Krishnan S (2011) Combining least-squares support vector machines for classification of biomedical signals: a case study with knee-joint vibroarthrographic signals. J Exp Theor Artif Intell 23(1):63–77
42. Wu Y, Shi L (2011) Analysis of altered gait rhythm in amyotrophic lateral sclerosis based on nonparametric probability density function estimation. Med Eng Phys 33(3):347–355
43. Wu Y, He J, Man Y, Arribas JI (2004) Neural network fusion strategies for identifying breast masses. In: Proceedings of 2004 international joint conference on neural networks, Budapest, pp 2437–2442
44. Wu Y, Wang C, Ng SC, Madabhushi A, Zhong Y (2006) Breast cancer diagnosis using neural-based linear fusion strategies. In: Proceedings of the 13th international conference on neural information processing, Hong Kong. LNCS, vol 4234, pp 165–175
45. Wu Y, Cai S, Yang S, Zheng F, Xiang N (2013) Classification of knee joint vibration signals using bivariate feature distribution estimation and maximal posterior probability decision criterion. Entropy 15(4):1375–1387
46. Yang S, Cai S, Zheng F, Wu Y, Liu K, Wu M, Zou Q, Chen J (2014) Representation of fluctuation features in pathologicalknee joint vibroarthrographic signals using kernel density modeling method. Med Eng Phys 36(10):1305–1311
47. Yang S, Zheng F, Luo X, Cai S, Wu Y, Liu K, Wu M, Chen J, Krishnan S (2014) Effective dysphonia detection using feature dimension reduction and kernel density estimation for patients with Parkinson's disease. PLoS One 9(2):e88825

Chapter 5
Summary and Research Directions

Abstract This chapter reviews the cutting-edge biomedical technologies for knee joint pathology diagnosis, and summarizes the major developments of knee joint vibroarthrographic signal analysis. The future research topics are also discussed in the conclusive text.

The knee is a very important joint that is composed of complex structures in the lower extremity. The knee flexion (with a slight medial and lateral rotation) and extension functions assist the human body to perform locomotion activities in daily life. However, the knee joint is very vulnerable to a variety of injuries and degenerative disorders. Common knee injuries include fractures, dislocations, sprains, tendon tears, ligament injuries, and meniscal tears [9]. In addition to physical trauma and misalignment, knee pain is usually caused by degeneration conditions for adults.

Osteoarthritis (OA) is a chronic inflammation of the entire knee joint involving the joint lining, ligaments, cartilage, and underlying bone. The degeneration and eventual breakdown of these tissues leads to knee pain and joint stiffness [2]. In United States, OA affects about 12.4 million (33.6 % population) of adults aged 65 years and older in 2005 [21]. In sense of statistical incidence, women have 45 % higher risk of incident knee OA than men, especially after 50 years old [22]. Effective diagnosis of articular cartilage degeneration and arthritis in the knee would increase more options for anti-inflammatory medication, physical therapy, and surgical treatment [26].

Nowadays, medical imaging techniques and arthroscopy have become prevailing in clinical diagnosis of knee osteo-arthropathy. Different imaging modalities have their particular radiographic characteristics and advantages summarized as follows.

Digital radiography modalities can improve the quality of X-ray images with slot and areal scanning modes than computed radiography systems. The digital radiography is more sensitive to high-density tissue calcification and mineral density of bones. Such a technique is good at detecting joint space narrowing, osteoporosis, and osteophytes based on X-ray images. The computed tomography can continuously rotate the X-ray tube during the scanning procedure, and then reconstruct the four-dimensional images from projections. The human body physiological dynamics and knee joint structures can be better visualized with multi-slice X-ray

© The Author(s) 2015
Y. Wu, *Knee Joint Vibroarthrographic Signal Processing and Analysis*,
SpringerBriefs in Bioengineering, DOI 10.1007/978-3-662-44284-5_5

computed tomography images than the digital radiography images. The common weakness of digital radiography and computed tomography modalities is that the status of soft tissues such as articular cartilage cannot be pictured with a direct appreciation, because the cartilage is not visible on X-ray images [5].

Ultrasonic instrumentation transmits ultrasonic pulses with a predefined frequency and bandwidth, and amplifies the received signal with a tradeoff between the penetration and resolution [7]. The higher frequency may provide ultrasonography images with a higher resolution, but the attenuation or penetration depth is lower. In clinical practice, cartilage thickness of OA patellas can be estimated with integrated reflection coefficient and apparent integrated backscatter within the frequency range of 20–60 MHz in B-mode ultrasonic imaging [6]. The integrated reflection coefficient variation reflects a change in acoustical impedance of the superficial layer of articular cartilages, which could indicate the fibrillation of the cartilage surface due to any disruption of collagen fibers [6]. The apparent integrated backscatter variation reflects the cartilage modifications in shape, according to the size and density of the scatterers in B-scan images [6].

Optical coherence tomography is a recently developed imaging technique that uses low-coherence interferometry near-infrared light to construct micrometer-resolution images within optical scattering tissues [19]. Similar to ultrasonography imaging, the optical coherence tomography is also limited by the penetration depth of infrared-based light photon. Based on the long wavelength light source, the optical coherence tomography modality can penetrate more deeply into the scattering tissue, but with a lower resolution. The tradeoff of penetration capability, resolution level, and better signal-to-noise ratio, is concerned for commercial optical coherence tomography modalities in clinical knee OA early detection.

Magnetic resonance imaging has been very popular for medical diagnosis of knee joint disorders and OA staging in the follow-up radiology examinations. Such a technique can prevent patients from exposure to ionizing radiation, and also can be used to investigate the anatomy (with diffusion weighted imaging or diffusion tensor imaging method) and physiology (with functional imaging method) of the human body [1]. The future development of medical imaging techniques for knee joint pathology examination would be the integration of multiple modalities toward a simultaneously functional and anatomical imaging with better spatial resolution. For example, the integration of positron emission tomography and magnetic resonance imaging can incorporate the magnetic resonance soft-tissue morphological imaging and the positron emission functional imaging in a single modality. The challenge is that the hybrid imaging modalities would require some special devices to balance tradeoffs between the performance of magnetic resonance tomography and the attenuation of positron emission tomography.

Knee arthroscopy has replaced the classic arthrotomy in knee pathology diagnosis and therapy [20]. An endoscope is used in a semi-invasive surgical procedure to inspect the join condition and treat meniscal tears through a small incision. Although such a well-established examination is referred to as the "gold standard" assessment method in orthopaedic practice, the effectiveness of knee arthroscopic surgery fairly depends on the operation skills and experience of the orthopaedic surgeons.

The arthroscopy is still invasive such that it is not well-suited for repeated assessments, because the same incision that undergos repeated surgical invasions is susceptible to bacterial infection.

Vibroarthrography is a burgeoning supplement technique for the detection of knee joint disorders [8]. The acceleration or acoustic signal emitted due to joint vibrations in the course of knee extension and flexion motions reflects the biomechanical characteristics of the knee [14]. The raw time series collected from the sensors should be properly conditioned by bandpass filters and preprocessed in order to remove the artifacts such as baseline wander, powerline interference, and random noise [3, 11, 29]. The signal preprocessing procedure is very important because the signal quality must be guaranteed prior to further analysis [26]. Decomposition and filtering are two types of VAG signal preprocessing methods. Filtering methods consider the frequency and statistical characteristics of signal and artifacts, so that the designed filters can enhance the signal or suppress the artifacts. Decomposition methods separate the signal and artifact components from the raw time series with different algorithms.

After the preprocessing procedure, a variety of signal processing approaches can be used to analyze the VAG signal features. Spatiotemporal and time-frequency analysis tools are frequently applied to study the joint time-frequency properties of VAG signals [4, 10, 12, 16, 23, 24, 30]. Recently, statistical methods have also been effectively employed in the VAG signal analysis [15]. Probability models were established for healthy normal and pathological VAG signals [17]. With the estimated probability density functions, the moments and other statistical parameters can be computed to describe the statistical features of articular degeneration. Fractal analysis and other nonlinear analysis algorithms are the state-of-the-art methods to reveal distinct chaotic dynamics and subtle fluctuations caused by osteoarthropathy or chondromalacia in the knee [18, 30].

Feature computing plays a pivotal role in VAG signal analysis as well. Correlation analysis tools are commonly implemented to study the mutual correlations between different features extracted from the artifact-free VAG signals. Feature selection and mapping methods can reduce the feature dimensions and increase the pattern diversity for further classifications. Kernel-based algorithms may project the signal scatters onto the nonlinear feature space for better pattern representations [30].

Plenty of computational intelligence techniques have been implemented for VAG signal pattern analysis. The state-of-the-art classification paradigms contain the Bayesian decision rule [28, 30], k-nearest neighbor algorithm [13], radial basis function network [15, 16], support vector machines [25], ensemble learning algorithms [4], and multiple classifier systems [27]. With the advanced computational methods, the accurate rate, sensitivity, specificity, and area under the receiver operating characteristic curve were greatly improved toward the clinical practice level.

Vibroarthrography has already shown its merits and potential in knee joint pathology detection and prognosis. In the future research, topics could focus on the distinct features of the pathological VAG signals related to particular knee joint disorders, such as chondromalacia, tears of meniscus, and so forth. Different digital signal processing methods can be used to study the time-variant complexity of VAG signals based on the biomechanical behaviors during knee flexion and extension motions. Localization of pathological area in the knee joint is also an interesting topic in the future work. Of course, more novel machine learning algorithms are also useful for dimensionality reduction and analysis of signal patterns. An effective computer-aided diagnosis system should be able to detect the types of knee inflammations, and stage the severity of disease as well.

References

1. Basser PJ, Jones DK (2002) Diffusion-tensor MRI: theory, experimental design and data analysis – a technical review. NMR Biomed 15(7):456–467
2. Bonnin M, Chambat P (2008) Osteoarthritis of the knee. Springer, New York
3. Cai S, Wu Y, Xiang N, Zhong Z, He J, Shi L, Xu F (2012) Detrending knee joint vibration signals with a cascade moving average filter. In: Proceedings of the 34th annual international conference of IEEE engineering in medicine and biology society, San Diego, pp 4357–4360
4. Cai S, Yang S, Zheng F, Lu M, Wu Y, Krishnan S (2013) Knee joint vibration signal analysis with matching pursuit decomposition and dynamic weighted classifier fusion. Comput Math Methods Med 2013:Article ID 904267
5. Carrillon Y (2008) Imaging knee osteoarthritis. In: Bonnin M, Chambat P (eds) Osteoarthritis of the knee. Springer, Paris, pp 3–14
6. Cherin E, Saied A, Laugier P, Netter P, Berger G (1998) Evaluation of acoustical parameter sensitivity to age-related and osteoarthritic changes in articular cartilage using 50-MHz ultrasound. Ultrasound Med Biol 24(3):341–354
7. Fenster A, Downey DB (1996) 3-D ultrasound imaging: a review. IEEE Eng Med Biol Mag 15(6):41–51
8. Frank CB, Rangayyan RM, Bell GD (1990) Analysis of knee sound signals for non-invasive diagnosis of cartilage pathology. IEEE Eng Med Biol Mag 9(1):65–68
9. Halpem B, Tucker L (2003) The knee crisis handbook. Rodale Books, Emmaus
10. Kim KS, Seo JH, Kang JU, Song CG (2009) An enhanced algorithm for knee joint sound classification using feature extraction based on time-frequency analysis. Comput Methods Programs Biomed 94(2):198–206
11. Krishnan S, Rangayyan RM (2000) Automatic de-noising of knee-joint vibration signals using adaptive time-frequency representations. Med Biol Eng Comput 38(8):2–8
12. Krishnan S, Rangayyan RM, Bell GD, Frank CB (2000) Adaptive time-frequency analysis of knee joint vibroarthrographic signals for noninvasive screening of articular cartilage pathology. IEEE Trans Biomed Eng 47(6):773–783
13. Liu K, Luo X, Zheng F, Yang S, Cai S, Wu Y (2014) Classification of knee joint vibroarthrographic signals using k-nearest neighbor algorithm. In: Proceedings of the 27th Canadian conference on electrical and computer engineering, Toronto, pp 150–153
14. Rangayyan RM (2002) Biomedical signal analysis: a case-study approach. IEEE/Wiley, New York
15. Rangayyan RM, Wu YF (2008) Screening of knee-joint vibroarthrographic signals using statistical parameters and radial basis functions. Med Biol Eng Comput 46(3):223–232
16. Rangayyan RM, Wu Y (2009) Analysis of vibroarthrographic signals with features related to signal variability and radial-basis functions. Ann Biomed Eng 37(1):156–163
17. Rangayyan RM, Wu Y (2010) Screening of knee-joint vibroarthrographic signals using probability density functions estimated with Parzen windows. Biomed Signal Process Control 5(1):53–58

18. Rangayyan RM, Oloumi F, Wu Y, Cai S (2013) Fractal analysis of knee-joint vibroarthrographic signals via power spectral analysis. Biomed Signal Process Control 8(1):26–29
19. Rashidifard C, Vercollone C, Martin S, Liu B, Brezinski ME (2013) The application of optical coherence tomography in musculoskeletal disease. Arthritis 2013:563268
20. Richmond JC, Bono JV, McKeon BP (2009) Knee arthroscopy. Springer, New York
21. Sacks JJ, Luo YH, Helmick CG (2010) Prevalence of specific types of arthritis and other rheumatic conditions in the ambulatory health care system in the United States. Arthritis Care Res 62(4):460–464
22. Srikanth VK, Fryer JL, Zhai G, Winzenberg TM, Hosmer D, Jones G (2005) A meta-analysis of sex difference prevalence, incidence and severity of osteoarthritis. Osteoarthr Cartil 13(9):769–781
23. Tanaka N, Hoshiyama M (2012) Vibroarthrography in patients with knee arthropathy. J Back Musculoskelet Rehabil 25(2):117–122
24. Wu Y, Krishnan S (2009) Classification of knee-joint vibroarthrographic signals using time-domain and time-frequency domain features and least-squares support vector machine. In: Proceedings of the 16th international conference on digital signal processing, Santorini, pp 361–366
25. Wu Y, Krishnan S (2011) Combining least-squares support vector machines for classification of biomedical signals: a case study with knee-joint vibroarthrographic signals. J Exp Theor Artif Intell 23(1):63–77
26. Wu Y, Krishnan S, Rangayyan RM (2010) Computer-aided diagnosis of knee-joint disorders via vibroarthrographic signal analysis: a review. Crit Rev Biomed Eng 38(2):201–224
27. Wu Y, Cai S, Lu M, Krishnan S (2011) An artificial-neural-network-based multiple classifier system for knee-joint vibration signal classification. In: Advances in computer, communication, control and automation. LNEE, vol 121. Springer, Berlin/Heidelberg, pp 235–242
28. Wu Y, Cai S, Yang S, Zheng F, Xiang N (2013) Classification of knee joint vibration signals using bivariate feature distribution estimation and maximal posterior probability decision criterion. Entropy 15(4):1375–1387
29. Wu Y, Yang S, Zheng F, Cai S, Lu M, Wu M (2014) Removal of artifacts in knee joint vibroarthrographic signals using ensemble empirical mode decomposition and detrended fluctuation analysis. Physiol Meas 35(3):429–439
30. Yang S, Cai S, Zheng F, Wu Y, Liu K, Wu M, Zou Q, Chen J (2014) Representation of fluctuation features in pathological knee joint vibroarthrographic signals using kernel density modeling method. Med Eng Phys 36(10):1305–1311